ISCHEMIC MYOCARDIUM AND ANTIANGINAL DRUGS

Perspectives in Cardiovascular Research
Volume 3

Perspectives in Cardiovascular Research

Series Editor:
Arnold M. Katz

Chief, Division of Cardiology
University of Connecticut School of Medicine
Farmington, Connecticut

Ischemic Myocardium and Antianginal Drugs

Perspectives in Cardiovascular Research
Volume 3

Editors

Martin M. Winbury, Ph.D.
Director
Pharmacological and Biological
* Evaluation*
Office of Scientific and Medical Affairs
Warner-Lambert Company
Morris Plains, New Jersey

Yasushi Abiko, M.D.
Professor of Pharmacology
Asahikawa Medical College
Asahikawa, Japan

Raven Press ■ New York

Raven Press, 1140 Avenue of the Americas, New York, New York 10036

Made in the United States of America

Library of Congress Cataloging in Publication Data
Main entry under title:

Ischemic myocardium and antianginal drugs.

  (Perspectives in cardiovascular research; v. 3)
  "Based on papers presented at the International
Symposium on Ischemic Myocardium and Antianginal Drugs
held at Asahikawa Medical College, Asahikawa, Japan,
September 25, 1978."
  Includes bibliographies and index.
  1. Coronary heart disease—Congresses.   2. Cardi-
ovascular agents—Congresses.   3.   Heart—Muscle—
Diseases—Congresses.   4.   Ischemia—Congresses.
I.   Winbury, Martin M.   II.   Abiko, Yasushi.
III.   International Symposium on Ischemic Myocardium and
Antianginal Drugs, Asahikawa, Japan, 1978.
RC685.C6I593   616.1'23'061   78–19618
ISBN 0–89004–380–9

Foreword

This volume is based on papers presented at the International Symposium on Ischemic Myocardium and Antianginal Agents held at Asahikawa Medical College, Asahikawa, Japan, as a satellite of the VIII Congress of Cardiology, Tokyo. Professor Yasushi Abiko was responsible for initiating the symposium, which was sponsored by the Department of Pharmacology, Asahikawa Medical College and the Asahikawa Medical Association. This was a fitting place for the symposium since Asahikawa is one of the newer medical colleges in Japan and the Department of Pharmacology, under Professor Abiko, has an interesting program on myocardial metabolism in the ischemic heart.

The purpose of the symposium was to bring together workers in the field of myocardial ischemia for a one-day intensive workshop with provocative discussion. Our objective was not to review what had been done by others in the past, but rather to have the participants report on new and exciting findings that have been developed recently. We were fortunate in having participants from a number of countries throughout the world, including Japan, West Germany, Iceland, South Africa, and the United States.

Professor Abiko and his associates at the Department of Pharmacology provided excellent arrangements for both the scientific and social portion of the symposium. The scientific sessions were enjoyed by all of the participants, particularly because of the informal nature and the challenging dialogue among the participants. Although there were many points of disagreement, which can be seen from the discussions, all of us felt that this workshop brought into focus new insights into the problem of the ischemic myocardium and enabled us to clarify a number of issues. Although many of us have participated in other programs on the ischemic myocardium and antianginal drugs, new perspectives on the subject were introduced at these sessions. The discussions not only clarified points that were made in the presentations but also brought out new concepts of particular importance, and the closing remarks of Lionel Opie succinctly summarized the presentations, providing an overview of the symposium.

Professor Abiko and his Department of Pharmacology, as well as all the other people from Asahikawa Medical College, deserve our thanks for making this meeting a wonderful experience.

Preface

This volume considers the ischemic myocardium from a physiological, phamacological, metabolic, and clinical viewpoint. Subjects range from ultrastructure, biophysics, intermediary metabolism, cyclic nucleotides, calcium antagonists, and therapy of coronary heart disease. The chapters are grouped into four main sections, as follows: "Structural and Biophysical Changes"; "Myocardial Blood Flow"; "Antianginal Drugs"; and "Metabolic Changes." At the conclusion of the volume, Dr. Lionel Opie, in his overview, gives a number of concluding remarks that cover the high points of the chapter and raises some additional questions. These remarks convey the general theme of each chapter in relation to the overall topic of the ischemic myocardium and antianginal drugs.

In the first main section ("Structural and Biophysical Changes"), J. Schaper et al. describe the ultrastructural changes produced by ischemia and the point of irreversibility. During ischemia, there is a fall in extracellular pH and (Ichihara et al.) and an increase in water permeability (Koyama et al.). Propranolol partially prevented the change in pH.

In the second section ("Myocardial Blood Flow"), it is shown that the vasodilator reserve of the inner regions—the endocardium—of the left ventricular wall is quite limited (Winbury and Howe). Comparison of the pharmacological profiles of various calcium antagonists indicates that there are distinctions between verapamil, nifedipine, and diltiazem (Ono and Hashimoto). This relates not only to vasodilator activity among various beds but to effects on the myocardium as well. In another chapter, Bing et al. demonstrate that dilitazem effectively counteracts some of the effects of acute ischemia on intermediary metabolism. This is due, in part, to the negative inotropic effect. Furthermore, the failure of mitonchondrial oxygen consumption and calcium binding seen on reperfusion is partially reversed by the drug. Both nitrates and beta-adrenergic blocking agents diminish the degree of myocardial ischemia in patients measured by biochemical markers, precordial EKG mapping, myocardial imaging, or ventricular angiograms (Bleifeld et al.). Coronary bypass surgery increases the coronary reserve and reduces the signs of coronary insufficiency.

Calcium antagonists are also considered in the section on antianginal drugs. Nakamura's group demonstrates that diltiazem prevents the ST segment elevation normally produced by acute ischemia; presumably this is a result of diminished cardiac work. In chronic ischemia, diltiazem increases subepicardial perfusion. Nifedipine, another calcium antagonist, is reported by Henry and Clark to protect the globally ischemic heart against contracture and calcium accumulation and to improve mechanical recovery after reperfusion. Nitroglycerin and beta-adrenergic blocking agents, but not potent coronary dilators or calcium antagonists, diminish the biochemical changes that normally occur with myocardial ischemia (Abiko et al.). The effect is probably indirect via a reduction in myocardial metabolism. W. Schaper describes a new model for study of therapeutic interventions on experimental acute myocardial infarction. The infarct size and area at risk are compared before and after treatment in the same dog.

Metabolic changes that accompany temporary ischemia and reperfusion are described by Imai et al. Ischemia produces rapid depletion of ATP and creatine phosphate and a cessation of contractility. Reperfusion permits good recovery of contractility, which is correlated with recovery of creatine phosphate but not ATP. Opie and Lubbe discuss experimental validation of their hypothesis linking accumulation of cAMP to the development of ventricular fibrillation shortly after the initiation of chronic ischemia. Interventions that produce a rise in cAMP levels in the isolated perfused rat heart increase the vulnerability to ventricular fibrillation induced by electrical stimulation during the vulnerable period. In another chapter, Gudbjarnason and Hallgrimsson show that, when rats are fed a diet of 10% cod liver oil, the normal 18]2n6 and 20:4n6 fatty acids are replaced by the longer and more unsaturated 22:6n3 fatty acid. These animals are more susceptible to isoproterenol stress than to norepinephrine stress. In humans with severe coronary atherosclerosis, the free fatty acid level of cardiac muscle is signficantly lower than in mild or moderate atherosclerosis.

Neely and associates report improved performance and reduced levels of acyl CoA in the ischemic regions of the dog and pig heart, but not in the rat heart. However, it may be that the beneficial effect is related to properties other than the change in acyl CoA.

Finally, in his overview, Opie introduces some questions and comments regarding the border zone between the normal and ischemic regions.

Martin M. Winbury

Acknowledgments

The editors of this volume would like to acknowledge with thanks the support of the following sponsors. Without their financial assistance, it would not have been possible to bring the participants together in Asahikawa.

Asahikawa Medical Association
Bayer Yakuhin, Ltd.
Chugai Pharmaceutical Co., Ltd.
Eisai Co., Ltd.
Funai Pharmaceutical Industries, Ltd.
Hoechst Japan, Ltd.
Dr. O. Kenmotsu, Department of Anesthesiology, Asahikawa Medical College
Kosugi Rika Co., Ltd.
Kyowa Hakko Kogyo Co., Ltd.
Mr. I. Matsumoto, Mayor of Asahikawa City
Mutoh Co., Ltd.
Nihon Kohden Kogyo Co., Ltd.
Nikkaki Co., Ltd.
Nippon C. H. Boehringer Sohn Co., Ltd.
Nissei Sangyo Co., Ltd.
Ono Pharmaceutical Co., Ltd.
Otsuka Pharmaceutical Company, Ltd.
Riko Shoji Co., Ltd.
Sandoz Yakuhin Co., Ltd.
San-Ei Instrument Co., Ltd.
Shimadzu Seisakusho, Ltd.
Shin Nihon Jitsugyo Co., Ltd.
Takeda Chemical Industries, Ltd.
Takeyama Co., Ltd.
Tanabe Seiyaku Co., Ltd.
Wako Pure Chemical Industries, Ltd.
Yamanouchi Pharmaceutical Co., Ltd.

Contents

Structural and Biophysical Changes

Myocardial Blood Flow

Antianginal Drugs

Metabolic Changes

Overview

Contributors

Yasushi Abiko*
Department of Pharmacology
Asahikawa Medical College
Asahikawa 078–11, Japan

Richard J. Bing*
Huntington Institute of Applied Medical
  Research and Huntington Memorial
  Hospital
Pasadena, California 91105
and
University of Southern California
Los Angeles, California 90023
and
California Institute of Technology
Pasadena, California 91109

W. Bleifeld*
Department of Cardiology
Medical Clinic II
University Hospital Eppendorf
D-2000 Hamburg, West Germany

Richard E. Clark
Cardiovascular Division
Department of Internal Medicine
Barnes Hospital
Washington University School of Medicine
St. Louis, Missouri 63110

David Garber
Department of Physiology
Milton S. Hershey Medical Center
Hershey, Pennsylvania 17033

Sigmundur Gudbjarnason*
Science Institute
University of Iceland
107 Reykjavik, Iceland

Jonas Hallgrimsson
Science Institute
University of Iceland
107 Reykjavik, Iceland

P. Hanrath
Department of Cardiology
Medical Clinic II
University Hospital Eppendorf
D-2000 Hamburg, West Germany

Koroku Hashimoto*
Hatano Research Institute
Food and Drug Safety Center
Kanagawa 257, Japan

Philip D. Henry*
Cardiovascular Division
Department of Internal Medicine
Barnes Hospital
Washington University School of Medicine
St. Louis, Missouri 63110

M. Hoffman
Department of Experimental Cardiology
Max-Planck-Institute for Physiological
  and Clinical Research
D-6350 Bad Nauheim, West Germany

Burton B. Howe
ICI—United States, Inc.
Wilmington, Delaware 19897

Kazuo Ichihara*
Department of Pharmacology
Asahikawa Medical College
Asahikawa 078–11, Japan

* These contributors participated in the International Symposium on Ischemic Myocardium and Antianginal Drugs, Asahikawa, Japan, September 25, 1978.

M. Ichihara
Department of Pharmacology
Asahikawa Medical College
Asahikawa 078–11, Japan

Jane Idell-Wenger
Department of Physiology
Milton S. Hershey Medical Center
Hershey, Pennsylvania 17033

Shoichi Imai*
Department of Pharmacology
Niigata University School of Medicine
Niigata 951, Japan

Takashi Izumi
Department of Pharmacology
Asahikawa Medical College
Asahikawa 078–11, Japan

Tomihiro Ikeo
Research Institute of Angiocardiology
and
Cardiovascular Clinic
Kyushu University Medical School
Fukuoka 812, Japan

Yoshihiro Kakiuchi
Research Institute of Applied Electricity
Hokkaido University
Sapporo 060, Japan

Hideo Kanaide
Research Institute of Angiocardiology
and
Cardiovascular Clinic
Kyushu University Medical School
Fukuoka 812, Japan

Yumi Katano
Department of Pharmacology
Niigata University School of Medicine
Niigata 951, Japan

Yuji Kikuchi
Research Institute of Applied Electricity
Hokkaido University
Sapporo 060, Japan

Yutaka Kikuchi
Research Institute of Angiocardiology
and
Cardiovascular Clinic
Kyushu University Medical School
Fukuoka 812, Japan

Yasushi Koiwaya
Research Institute of Angiocardiology
and
Cardiovascular Clinic
Kyushu University Medical School
Fukuoka 812, Japan

Tomiyasu Koyama*
Research Institute of Applied Electricity
Hokkaido University
Sapporo 060, Japan

W. Kupper
Department of Cardiology
Medical Clinic II
University Hospital Eppendorf
D-2000 Hamburg, West Germany

W. F. Lubbe
Green Lane Hospital
Auckland 3, New Zealand

D. Mathey
Department of Cardiology
Medical Clinic II
University Hospital Eppendorf
D-2000 Hamburg, West Germany

Kathleen McDonough
Department of Physiology
Milton S. Hershey Medical Center
Hershey, Pennsylvania 17033

Michitaka Mori
Research Institute of Angiocardiology
and
Cardiovascular Clinic
Kyushu University Medical School
Fukuoka 812, Japan

Motoomi Nakamura*
Research Institute of Angiocardiology
and
Cardiovascular Clinic
Kyushu University Medical School
Fukuoka 812, Japan

James R. Neely
Department of Physiology
Milton S. Hershey Medical Center
Hershey, Pennsylvania 17033

Hiroshi Ono
Hatano Research Institute
Food and Drug Safety Center
Kanagawa 257, Japan

Lionel H. Opie*
MRC Ischaemic Heart Disease Research
 Unit
Department of Medicine
Groote Schuur Hospital
and
University of Cape Town Medical School
7925 Cape Town, South Africa

S. Pasyk
Department of Experimental Cardiology
Max-Planck-Institute for Physiological
 and Clinical Research
D-6350 Bad Nauheim, West Germany

Günter Pawlik
Huntington Institute of Applied Medical
 Research
and
Huntington Memorial Hospital
Pasadena, California 91105

Angelika Rackl
Huntington Institute of Applied Medical
 Research
and
Huntington Memorial Hospital
Pasadena, California 91105

Ken Sakai
Department of Pharmacology
Niigata University School of Medicine
Niigata 951, Japan

Jutta Schaper*
Department of Experimental Cardiology
Max-Planck-Institute for Physiological
 and Clinical Research
D-6350 Bad Nauheim, West Germany

Wolfgang Schaper*
Department of Experimental Cardiology
Max-Planck-Institute for Physiological
 and Clinical Research
D-6350 Bad Nauheim, West Germany

Yutaka Senda
Research Institute of Angiocardiology
and
Cardiovascular Clinic
Kyushu University Medical School
Fukuoka 812, Japan

Norio Shimamoto
Department of Pharmacology
Niigata University School of Medicine
Niigata 951, Japan

Kenji Sunagawa
Research Institute of Angiocardiology
and
Cardiovascular Clinic
Kyushu University Medical School
Fukuoka 812, Japan

Ronald Weishaar
Huntington Institute of Applied Medical
 Research
and
Huntington Memorial Hospital
Pasadena, California 91105

Martin M. Winbury*
Office of Scientific and Medical Affairs
Warner-Lambert Company
Morris Plains, New Jersey 07950

Akira Yamada
Research Institute of Angiocardiology
and
Cardiovascular Clinic
Kyushu University Medical School
Fukuoka 812, Japan

Structural and Biophysical Changes

Ischemic Myocardium and Antianginal Drugs,
edited by M. M. Winbury and Y. Abiko.
Raven Press, New York © 1979.

Early Ultrastructural Changes in Myocardial Ischemia and Infarction

Jutta Schaper, S. Pasyk, M. Hofmann, and W. Schaper

Department of Experimental Cardiology, Max-Planck-Institute for Physiological and Clinical Research, D-6350 Bad Nauheim, West Germany

The mode of structural development of myocardial infarction is largely unknown. Although numerous studies have examined various stages of regional myocardial ischemia, a systematic evaluation of ultrastructural changes is lacking. The electron microscope is the ideal tool for this kind of investigation because light microscopy and histochemistry are too insensitive to record the structural changes that occur within the first hours of coronary occlusion. We undertook the present study (a) to investigate the alterations of the cardiac cells that occur with respect to time after coronary occlusion; and (b) to determine the "point of no return" in cellular ischemic injury.

MATERIALS AND METHODS

Experimental Procedure

Fifteen mongrel dogs of either sex weighing about 20 kg were anesthetized, and their chests were opened at the fifth intercostal space under artificial respiration. The heart was suspended in a pericardial cradle; after a hemodynamic steady state was reached, the left anterior descending coronary artery (LAD) was occluded by ligature. After 45 min ($n = 6$) or 90 min ($n = 6$), the ligature was released and blood flow through the LAD was reestablished. The chests were then closed, and the animals were allowed to recover for 48 hr. In a third group of dogs ($n = 3$), the occlusion of the LAD was continued for 48 hr. Thereafter, all dogs (from all three groups) were sacrificed by an overdose of pentobarbital sodium. The hearts were removed from the thorax, cut into slices, and incubated in a tetrazolium solution (7) for macroscopic determination of the size and localization of the infarct.

Electron Microscopy

Cardiac biopsies were taken from the beating hearts using a Tru-cut® biopsy needle (Travenol). The biopsies were taken from the center of the ischemic area, which could be identified by its purple-blue color and by the fact that this part of the myocardium did not contract. Biopsies were taken either at the end of the ischemic interval or at the beginning of the reperfusion period (15 min after release of the ligature). The biopsy procedure yielded transmural tissue cylinders that were divided into endocardial, endomural, and epicardial tissue samples. The tissue was immediately fixed in cold 3% glutaraldehyde buffered with 0.1 M cacodylate at a pH of 7.4. After the tissue was thoroughly rinsed in cacodylate, it was postfixed in OsO_4 buffered with veronal acetate, dehydrated in a graded series of ethanol, treated with propylene oxide, and embedded in Epon®. Semithin sections (1 to 2 μm thick) were cut and stained with toluidine blue. After selection of artifact-free areas, thin sections (600 Å) were prepared, stained with uranyl acetate and lead citrate, and viewed in a Philips EM 300 electron microscope.

RESULTS

In order to avoid artifacts (originating from faulty preparation of the tissue), biopsies from normal canine hearts were also investigated electron microscopically. These tissue samples showed a completely normal ultrastructure.

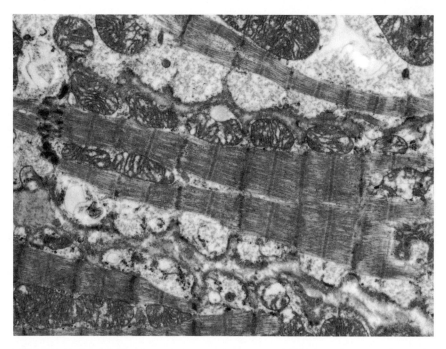

FIG. 1. After 45 min of ischemia, most myocardial cells are moderately damaged. Intracellular edema is evident. ×14,900.

Forty-Five Minutes of Ischemia

At the end of the ischemic interval, the majority of subendocardial cells were moderately damaged; however, some severely damaged and some irreversibly injured cells were also observed. Myocardial cell injury included mitochondrial matrix clearing, loss of normal dense granules, and fragmentation of some cristae. In the irreversibly injured cells, large amorphous densities within the matrical space of the mitochondria were present. The nuclei either exhibited no change or showed swelling with margination of chromatin. Most sarcomeres were in contraction; contracture bands were occasionally present. Intracellular edema was a regular finding. All other cell organelles appeared unchanged (Fig. 1). The interstitial space contained fluid and protein-like substances; sometimes red blood cells were also observed. Small blood vessels, however, were normal (Fig. 2).

Subepicardial tissue samples showed an almost normal ultrastructure, except for the occasional absence of the normal dense granules from the mitochondria and the occurrence of a slight intracellular edema (Fig. 3).

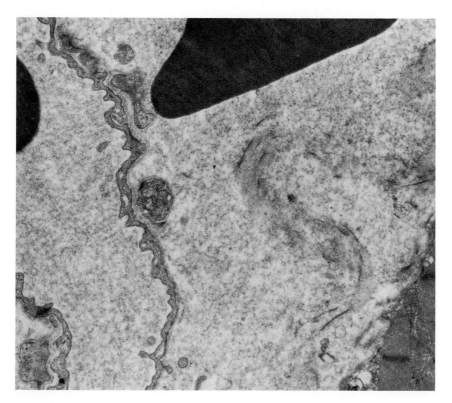

FIG. 2. At the end of 45 min of ischemia, fluid, protein, and red blood cells are present in the extravascular space. ×10,700.

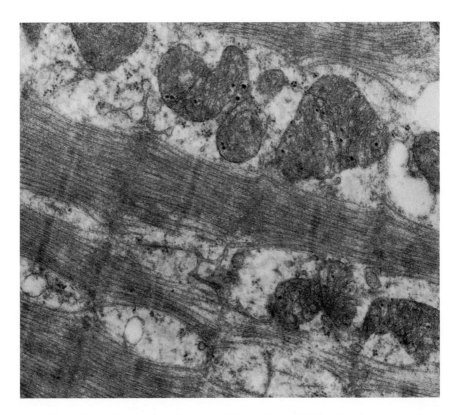

FIG. 3. After 45 min of ischemia, subepicardial tissue shows slightly altered mitochondria and intracellular edema. ×18,400.

After 45 min of occlusion plus 15 min of reperfusion, the entire tissue sample from the subendocardium showed more severe damage than after ischemia alone. Many of the cells were irreversibly damaged (destroyed mitochondria showed large amorphous densities, and pronounced swelling of the nuclei was evident). All cells exhibited numerous prominent contracture bands (Fig. 4). The subepicardial tissue showed persisting slight intracellular edema, whereas all cellular components appeared normal.

The presence of fluid, protein-like substances, and erythrocytes in the interstitial space of the subendocardial sample was more pronounced after 45 min of occlusion and 15 min of reperfusion than after the ischemic interval alone; the subepicardial tissue lacked any such signs.

In conclusion, 45 min of regional ischemia caused variable cellular injury ranging from moderate to irreversible in the subendocardial layer; that is, most cells were ischemic and some were already necrotic. Cardiac tissue from the subepicardium showed only slight changes that receded upon reperfusion. After restoration of blood flow, many cells were irreversibly injured, but others showed

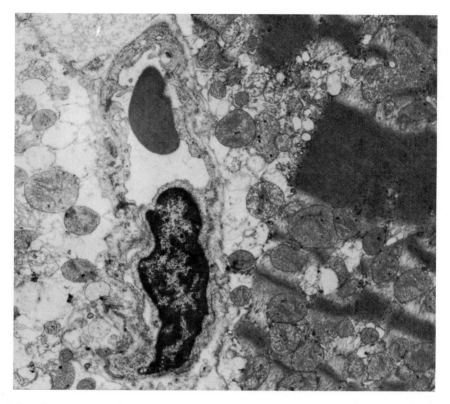

FIG. 4. On reperfusion after 45 min of ischemia, irreversible injury is present in many myocytes. Note the contraction band at the *right upper corner.* ×13,200.

improvement of their ultrastructure. Although extravasation of fluid, protein, and erythrocytes was present after ischemia alone, it was much more pronounced after reperfusion had been initiated.

Ninety Minutes of Ischemia

At the end of the ischemic interval, many cells of the subendocardial tissue were moderately or severely injured (swollen mitochondria, fragmentation of cristae, swelling of the nuclei, and some contracture bands were evident). In contrast to the tissue samples subjected to the shorter ischemic interval, these cells usually exhibited a large number of fat droplets. These droplets were of moderate density and lacked a limiting membrane (Fig. 5).

Irreversibly injured cells showed a partial loss of the cell membrane and extremely cleared mitochondria; these contained only a few cristae, but large amorphous densities (Fig. 6). Some mitochondria were condensed into electron-dense patches, and others were disintegrating into small membranous particles.

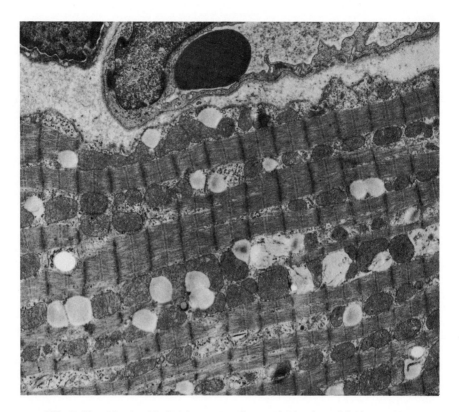

FIG. 5. After 90 min of ischemia many cells contain droplets of lipids. ×7,200.

The nuclei showed swelling or shrinkage. Whereas the sarcomeres were contracted in moderately injured cells, they were disrupted, hypercontracted, or
completely relaxed in irreversibly damaged myocardial cells.

The cells from the subepicardial tissue showed slight to moderate injury (the
mitochondria exhibited loss of normal dense granules, clearing of the matrix,
and some fragmentation of cristae; slight swelling of the nuclei was evident).
Intracellular edema was present (Fig. 7).

The interstitial space was of normal appearance in the subepicardium, but
in the subendocardium it contained fluid, protein-like substances, fibrin, erythrocytes, and neutrophil granulocytes (PMN). The latter were either intact or disintegrating, and they were seen to adhere to irreversibly damaged myocytes (Figs.
6 and 8). Macrophages invaded the space between myocardial cells. They contained lysosomes, phagosomes, and numerous elements of proliferating rough
endoplasmic reticulum. The endothelium of many small blood vessels was swollen, but other capillaries and venules were completely normal.

After reperfusion, more cells in the subendocardial layer were irreversibly
injured than after ischemia alone. The mitochondria showed clearing, loss of

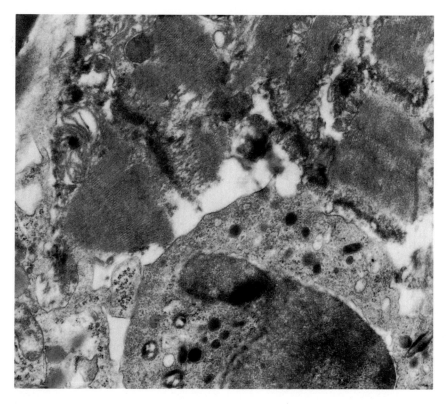

FIG. 6. Many cells are irreversibly injured after 90 min of ischemia. A neutrophil granulocyte penetrates the myocardial cell. ×16,800.

cristae, and many large amorphous densities. The nuclei usually showed shrinkage. The sarcomeres were disorganized or hypercontracted, resulting in contracture bands. The sarcolemma was frequently interrupted (Fig. 9). There were also cells that showed a partial reversal to normal of their ischemic alterations.

The subepicardial tissue showed improvement of the subcellular integrity. The interstitial space of the subepicardium was of normal appearance, but the extravascular space in the subendocardial layer contained platelets and monocytes in addition to fluid and the formed elements of the blood mentioned above. Many PMNs and a few macrophages adhered closely to the irreversibly injured cells or invaded them. The capillaries and venules frequently showed a very thin wall with numerous membranous blebs, or the endothelium was swollen. Blood vessels that appeared normal usually contained erythrocytes. Microthrombi consisting of erythrocytes and platelets were seen to occlude the vascular lumen (Fig. 10).

In conclusion, 90 min of ischemia caused both severe and irreversible injury in subendocardial cells; i.e., the cells were either ischemic or already necrotic.

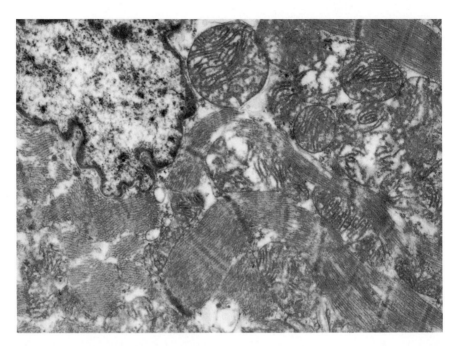

FIG. 7. Subepicardial tissue 90 min after ischemia shows moderate ischemic injury. Note the slight swelling of the nucleus. ×18,500.

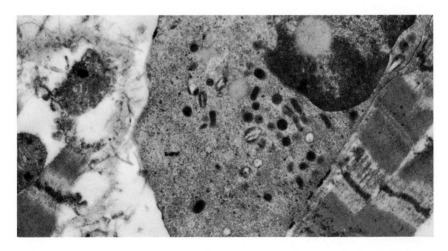

FIG. 8. A neutrophil granulocyte is closely adhering to a myocardial cell (90 min of ischemia). ×15,200.

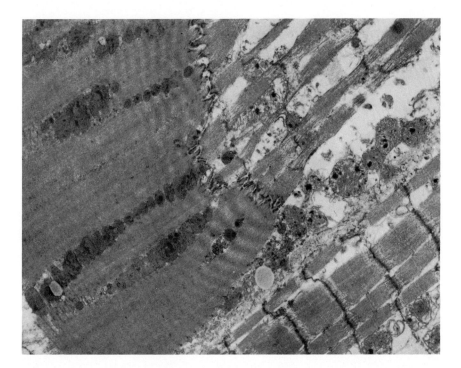

FIG. 9. Irreversibly injured myocardial cells after 90 min of ischemia plus reperfusion. The mitochondria contain large amorphous densities; an area of contracture is seen at the *left*. ×7,200.

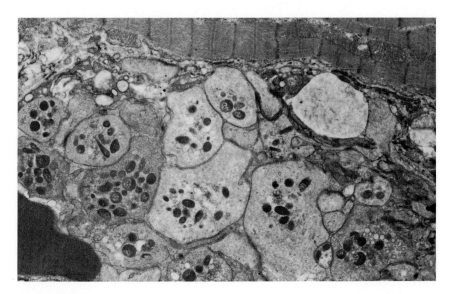

FIG. 10. Numerous platelets occlude the lumen of a small blood vessel (90 min ischemia and reperfusion). ×7,200.

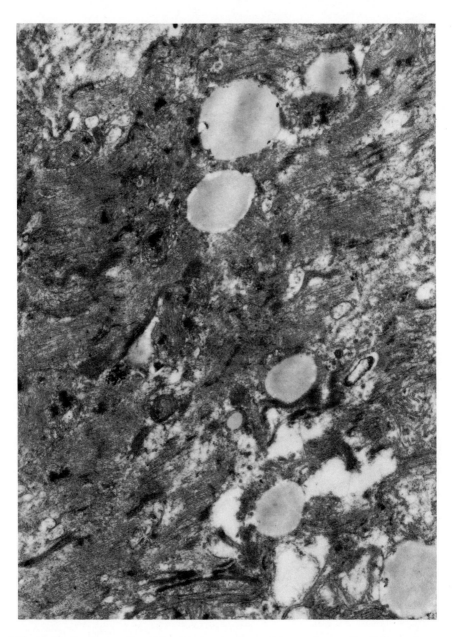

FIG. 11. Cardiac tissue after 48 hr of ischemia shows disintegration of all cellular structures. ×20,400.

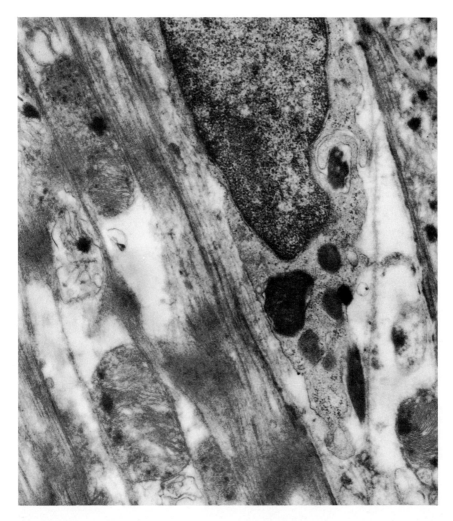

FIG. 12. A macrophage penetrates between two myocardial cells that are irreversibly damaged (48 hr of ischemia). A persisting basement membrane delineates the original size of the myocyte. ×22,400.

Necrotic cells were more frequent after 90 min than after 45 min of ischemia. Although reperfusion increased the number of necrotic cells, other cells showed structural recovery.

Permanent Occlusion (48 hr)

After 48 hr of regional ischemia, all myocardial cells were destroyed. The sarcolemma was disrupted. The mitochondria were strongly condensed or extremely electron lucent, showing many large amorphous densities, or broken up into small membranous particles. The nuclei showed either extreme swelling or shrinkage. The sarcomeres were condensed, forming contraction bands, or they were distorted and were starting to dissolve at the I-bands. In many cases, only parts of the myocytes were still present, and only the course of the still-persisting basement membrane indicated the original size of the cell. Erythrocytes, neutrophil granulocytes (mostly disintegrating), platelets and monocytes, macrophages, and plasma protein were observed between these remnants of myocardial cells. Most capillaries and venules were destroyed; a few contained erythrocytes, and these were of normal appearance (Figs. 11 and 12).

In conclusion, after permanent coronary occlusion for 48 hr, the myocardial cells not only are irreversibly injured but are already destroyed and partly removed by the action of neutrophil granulocytes and phagocytic cells.

DISCUSSION

Progression with Time of Ultrastructural Ischemic Changes

The fact that the severity of ischemic injury increases with time has been thoroughly established in global ischemia of the heart (1,12,13,15). Despite the specific differences between global and regional ischemia (6,9), the same principle apparently is true in the latter experimental model. Progression of cellular injury can be observed in reversibly injured cells as well as in irreversibly damaged myocytes. Progression of damage in reversible injury consists of increasing clearing of the mitochondrial matrix and fragmentation and loss of cristae. The nuclei show signs of injury only at later stages; i.e., they are apparently more resistant to lack of oxygen than are the mitochondria. The irreversibly injured (necrotic) cells also show a progression of cellular changes. At later stages, the mitochondria exhibit loss of the outer membrane, which results either in "giant mitochondria" (originating from several fused mitochondria) or in mitochondrial "debris" consisting of small membranous particles. However, when the mitochondria are already disintegrating, most nuclei are still intact although they are swollen or shrunken. Destruction of the sarcomeres also progresses with time; the sarcolemma becomes disrupted at later phases of injury. All these phenomena may be reduced to one common denominator—disturbances of the integrity of all membranous parts of the cell. Although the central event that transforms reversible into irreversible injury is unknown, there is much evidence to prove that disturbances in cellular membrane properties are very important factors (2,4,14).

Reperfusion after a certain period of ischemia apparently has two different effects on ischemic cells: (a) Reperfusion most probably accelerates cellular injury that would otherwise become evident after several hours of ischemia; i.e., it changes ischemic cells into necrotic cells (this may be an additional argument for a latent crucial disturbance of membrane functions). (b) Reperfusion causes the structural recovery of many cells in the ischemic subendocardium and of all cells (except after permanent occlusion) in the subepicardial layer. Both these facts may indicate that the ultrastructural criteria for judgment of the severity of injury are not completely reliable when tissue obtained at the end of the ischemic period is investigated. Tissue samples obtained during reperfusion may reflect a picture nearer to the true conditions. The variable severity of ischemic injury within one tissue sample may have been caused by persisting but insufficient collateral flow. It has been shown (11) that in the center of ischemic myocardium, due to collateral blood flow, about 10% of the normal myocardial perfusion rate is still present. This residual flow most probably is unequally distributed. Some cells, therefore, may be more severely deprived of oxygen than others.

The accumulation of triglycerides may be the morphological equivalent of changes in cardiac metabolism caused by a low perfusion rate. In hearts sufficiently supplied with oxygen, fatty acids (from the breakdown of triglycerides) are the main fuel for energy production (6). When oxygen supply is insufficient, only glucose can be used, and triglycerides are stored within the cells. Most probably, the persisting low-flow condition due to collateral flow is also responsible for the emigration of blood components. Although unable to maintain aerobic metabolism (as indicated by the accumulation of triglycerides and the destruction of the cellular ultrastructure), this residual flow makes the exudation of fluid and corpuscular blood elements possible. The presence of neutrophil granulocytes adhering closely to severely injured myocardial cells indicates that the effects of ischemia were aggravated by a nonspecific inflammatory reaction.

It may be hypothesized that the ischemic myocardial cells release a factor that alters vascular permeability (16) and mediates stickiness (3), chemotaxis, and chemokinesis (8) of the neutrophils. One factor possibly involved in increasing vascular permeability may be histamine (5); other substances, such as bradykinin, prostaglandins, or cyclic AMP, or the altered conditions of low pH and low pO_2 or raised pCO_2 may also play a role in causing this inflammatory reaction.

The "Point of No Return" in Cellular Injury

The definition of irreversibility implies the inability of the tissue to recover from the noxious condition after the noxious condition has been removed (in regional ischemia, after the lack of blood has been removed by reperfusion). Thus, cells that do not recover from injury are past the "point of no return." From this study, it is evident that 45 min of ischemia may already cause irreversible injury to some cells and that after 90 min of ischemia, myocardial injury has proceeded significantly.

It is difficult, however, to define a certain time interval after which ischemia results in cellular necrosis for the following reason: It has been shown that the size of myocardial infarction—i.e., the number of irreversibly injured cells— depends not only on time but also on the amount of residual blood flow available to the ischemic area by collaterals and on the rate of oxygen consumption (10). Therefore, time is only one among three variables. In the experiments described here, oxygen consumption was relatively high and collateral perfusion was low. Under these conditions, subendocardial infarction was already partially present after 45 min of ischemia. Myocardial infarction was greater after 90 min of ischemia (as evaluated by macroscopic histochemistry), which means that more cells were past the "point of no return" than after a shorter interval. The infarcted area was even larger after permanent occlusion for 48 hr; i.e., irreversible injury leading to cellular necrosis occurred in an increasing number of cells and it also affected the subepicardial tissue layer that had shown structural recovery after shorter periods of ischemia.

REFERENCES

1. Bretschneider, H. J. (1964): Überlebens- und Wiederbelebungszeit des herzens bei Normo- und Hypothermie. *Verh. Dtsch. Ges. Kreislaufforsch,* 30:11–34.
2. Decker, R. S., Poole, A. R., Griffin, E. E., Dingle, J. T., and Wildenthal, K. (1977): Altered distribution of lysosomal cathepsin D in ischemic myocardium. *J. Clin. Invest.,* 59:911–921.
3. Grant, L. (1973): The sticking and emigration of white blood cells in inflammation. In: *The Inflammatory Process, Volume 2,* edited by B. M. Zweifach, L. Grant, and R. T. McCluskey, pp. 205–244. Academic Press, New York.
4. Jennings, R. B. (1976): Relationship of acute ischemia to functional defects and irreversibility. *Circulation (Suppl. I),* 53:I-26–I-29.
5. Majno, G., Shea, S. M., and Leventhal, M. (1969): Endothelial contraction induced by histamine-type mediators. An electron microscopic study. *J. Cell Biol.,* 42:647–672.
6. Opie, L. (1976): Effects of regional ischemia on metabolism of glucose and fatty acids. Relative rates of aerobic and anaerobic energy production during myocardial infarction and comparison with effects of anoxia. *Circ. Res. (Suppl. I),* 38:I-52–I-74.
7. Pearse, E. G. E. (1972): *Histochemistry. Theoretical and Applied, Volume 2.* Churchill Livingstone, Edinburgh.
8. Ramsey, W. S., and Grant, L. (1973): Chemotaxis. In: *The Inflammatory Process, Volume 1,* edited by B. M. Zweifach, L. Grant, and R. T. McCluskey, pp. 287–362. Academic Press, New York.
9. Schaper, J. (1978): Ultrastructural characteristics in regional versus global ischemia. *J. Mol. Cell. Cardiol.,* 10:95.
10. Schaper, W., Carl, M., and Hort, W. (1977): Evolution of infarcts with time after experimental coronary occlusion. *Circulation (Suppl. III),* 56:III-138.
11. Schaper, W., Flameng, W., Winkler, B., Wüsten, B., Türschmann, W., Neugebauer, G., and Carl, M. (1976): Quantification of collateral resistance in acute and chronic experimental coronary occlusion in the dog. *Circ. Res.,* 39:371–377.
12. Schaper, J., Hehrlein, F., Schlepper, M., and Thiedemann, K.-U. (1977): Ultrastructural alterations during ischemia and reperfusion in human hearts during cardiac surgery. *J. Mol. Cell. Cardiol.,* 9:175–190.
13. Stemmer, E. A., McCart, P., Stanton, W. W., Thibault, W., Dearden, L. S., and Conolly, J. E. (1973): Functional and structural alterations in the myocardium during aortic cross-clamping. *J. Thorac. Cardiovasc. Surg.,* 66:754–770.
14. Trump, B. F., Mergner, W., Kaling, M. W., and Saladina, A. J. (1976): Studies on the subcellular pathophysiology of ischemia. *Circulation (Suppl. I),* 53:I-17–I-26.
15. Tyers, G. F. O., Williams, E. H., Hughes, H. C., and Todd, G. J. (1977): Effect of perfusate temperature on myocardial protection from ischemia. *J. Thorac. Cardiovasc. Surg.,* 73:766–781.
16. Willoughby, D. A. (1973): Mediation of increased vascular permeability in inflammation. In: *The Inflammatory Process, Volume 2,* edited by B. M. Zweifach, L. Grant, and R. T. McCluskey, pp. 303–329. Academic Press, New York.

Ischemic Myocardium and Antianginal Drugs,
edited by M. M. Winbury and Y. Abiko.
Raven Press, New York © 1979.

Possible Role of Beta-Adrenergic Receptors in Myocardial Metabolic Response to Ischemia

K. Ichihara, M. Ichihara, and Y. Abiko

Department of Pharmacology, Asahikawa Medical College, Asahikawa 078-11, Japan

It is generally accepted that lack of oxygen supply to the myocardial cells shifts the pattern of myocardial metabolism from aerobic to anaerobic (3,13,15). We have demonstrated that coronary artery ligation causes acceleration of glycogenolysis and accumulation of the intermediates of glycolysis in the ischemic region of the myocardium, and that response to ischemia of the endocardial layers is more prominent than that of the epicardial layers (8). We have also demonstrated that myocardial pH measured by a pH microelectrode decreases markedly during coronary artery ligation (9).

Several investigators have proposed that beta-adrenergic receptors play an important role in the acceleration of anaerobic metabolism during myocardial ischemia (12,19); i.e., the acceleration of anaerobic metabolism during ischemia occurs as a result of the release of catecholamines from stored sites in the myocardium. Dobson and Mayer (4) and Wollenberger et al. (20) reported that the metabolic response to ischemia was virtually abolished by beta-adrenergic blockers, and Wollenberger and Shahab (21) also found in isolated perfused rat and rabbit hearts that the level of norepinephrine in the perfusate increased during oxygen deprivation.

The present study, therefore, was undertaken to examine the effect of beta-adrenergic blockers on the stimulation of anaerobic metabolism and the decrease in myocardial pH caused by coronary artery ligation in order to investigate the possibility that beta-adrenergic receptors are involved in the mechanism of anaerobic response of the myocardium to ischemia.

METHODS

Two groups of mongrel dogs of either sex were employed. One group was used to examine the effect of pretreatment with beta blockers (propranolol or carteolol) on metabolic response to ischemia (metabolic experiment); and the second was used to examine the effect of propranolol on ischemia-induced decrease in myocardial pH (pH experiment). The dogs in the pH experiment group were further divided into two subgroups. In the first subgroup, changes in the myocardial pH after coronary artery ligation in the presence or absence of propranolol were investigated; and in the second subgroup, changes in the myocardial pH after beta-adrenergic stimulant injection in the presence or absence of propranolol were investigated.

Animal Preparation

The dogs were anesthetized with sodium pentobarbital (30 mg/kg, i.v.), and the left side of the thorax was opened to permit free access to the left ventricular myocardium. One of the small branches of the left anterior descending coronary artery was dissected free from the adjacent tissue and a silk thread was placed around the branch for ligation. A metal cannula was introduced into the right femoral vein for intravenous injections. Arterial blood pressure was measured with an electronic manometer, and heart rate was counted from the electrocardiogram (limb lead II).

Procedure for Metabolic Experiment

Saline, propranolol (1 mg/kg), or carteolol (10 µg/kg) was injected intravenously over a period of 30 sec; 5 min after the start of each injection, the small branch of the coronary artery was ligated. Immediately before or 1.5, 3, 7, or 30 min after coronary artery ligation, the region supplied by the ligated coronary artery was rapidly removed with scissors and immediately pressed and frozen with freezing clamps previously chilled with liquid nitrogen (Fig. 1). The frozen and pressed sample was placed on a block of dry ice and carefully cracked into fragments with a chisel that had been chilled with liquid nitrogen so that the fragments originating in the endocardial layers and those in the epicardial layers could be collected separately. Each of the endo- and epicardial frozen tissue samples (fragments) was divided into three samples. The first samples were weighed (100 to 150 mg) and analyzed for glycogen content according to the method of Seifter et al. (17). The second samples were weighed (300 to 500 mg) and extracted to determine the glucose-1-phosphate (G1P), glucose-

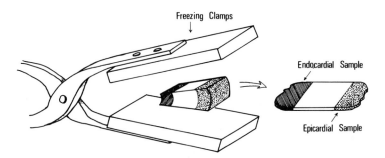

FIG. 1. Schematic illustration of a method for obtaining frozen endo- and epicardial samples. (From Ichihara et al., ref. 8, with permission.)

6-phosphate (G6P), fructose-6-phosphate (F6P), pyruvate, and lactate contents. The content in the samples of the intermediates listed above was measured in neutralized perchloric acid extract according to the standard enzymatic procedure (2), but the lactate content was measured colorimetrically according to the method of Barker and Summerson (1). The third samples were weighed (200 to 350 mg) and extracted to determine the activity of the phosphorylase. The activity of phosphorylase was assayed by measuring the inorganic phosphate (P_i) released as a result of adding G1P to a mixture that contained tissue glycerol extract and the phosphorylase assay medium described in a previous paper (8). P_i was measured according to the method of Fiske and Subbarow (5). The activity of phosphorylase a + b (total phosphorylase) was assayed in the presence of 5′-adenosine monophosphate (5′-AMP), and that of phosphorylase a was assayed in the absence of 5′-AMP.

Procedure for pH Experiment

A glass pH microelectrode (MI-408A, Microelectrode, Inc.) was inserted into the region of the left ventricle that was expected to become ischemic when the coronary artery was ligated; the tip of the pH electrode was placed about 6 mm below the surface of the myocardium. The electrode was suspended by a spring from a support so as to move with the beating of the heart. The reference electrode was attached to the thoracic wall. The pH and reference electrodes were connected to the pH meter and calibrated with standard pH solution (pH 6.30 and pH 7.38). Changes in myocardial pH before and after coronary artery ligation, after release of coronary ligation, and after the injection of isoproterenol (0.3 μg/kg) were recorded continuously with a pen recorder. Propranolol (1 mg/kg) was injected intravenously about 10 min before coronary artery ligation or isoproterenol injection.

Statistical Analysis

All values are expressed as mean ± SE. Statistical significance was assumed when a *p* value of 0.05 or less was obtained.

RESULTS

Glycogenolysis and Beta Blockers in Ischemic Myocardium

Changes in the glycogen level and phosphorylase activity in the endo- and epicardial layers after coronary artery ligation in the presence or absence of propranolol and carteolol are illustrated in Fig. 2.

In saline-pretreated dogs, before coronary artery ligation, the endocardial glycogen level (11.04 ± 0.75 mg/g) and total phosphorylase (16.6 ± 0.5 μmoles released P_i/g/min) and phosphorylase a activity (5.0 ± 0.5 μmoles released

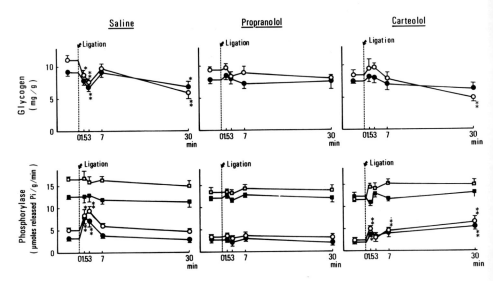

FIG. 2. Effect of beta-adrenergic blockers on changes in endo- and epicardial glycogen *(upper panel)* and phosphorylase activity *(lower panel)* caused by coronary artery ligation. A small branch of the left anterior descending coronary artery was ligated at 0 min. Saline, propranolol (1 mg/kg), or carteolol (10 μg/kg) was injected intravenously 5 min before coronary artery ligation. The ischemic region of the myocardium supplied by the ligated coronary artery was removed immediately before or 1.5, 3, 7, or 30 min after coronary artery ligation. Total phosphorylase (phosphorylase a + b) activity *(squares)* was assayed with 5'-AMP and phosphorylase a activity *(circles)* without 5'-AMP. Each point and bar represents mean ± SE. Asterisks denote significance of difference from preligation value (*, $p < 0.05$; ⁑, $p < 0.01$). *Open symbols* denote endocardial layers; *solid symbols* denote epicardial layers. (Adapted from data in ref. 8.)

$P_i/g/min$) were significantly higher ($p < 0.05$) than the epicardial (9.24 ± 0.6 mg/g and 12.6 ± 0.3 and 3.2 ± 0.4 μmoles released $P_i/g/min$, respectively). Immediately after coronary artery ligation, the activity of phosphorylase a increased with the decrease of the glycogen level. The total phosphorylase activity, however, did not change appreciably. It is likely that coronary artery ligation produces conversion of phosphorylase from b-form to a-form. Coronary artery ligation for 3 min increased the activity of the phosphorylase a as much as twofold and decreased the level of glycogen to about 70% of its initial level. This result is in accord with the view that myocardial glycogenolysis is accelerated during oxygen deprivation.

In propranolol-pretreated dogs, the endo- and epicardial glycogen levels (9.33 ± 0.40 and 7.83 ± 0.55 mg/g, respectively) and phosphorylase a activities (3.3 ± 0.2 and 2.7 ± 0.5 μmoles released $P_i/g/min$, respectively) before coronary artery ligation were slightly low compared with those obtained in saline-pretreated dogs. Pretreatment with propranolol inhibited completely the changes in the glycogen level and phosphorylase a activity of both layers caused by coronary artery ligation.

In carteolol-pretreated dogs, the endo- and epicardial glycogen levels (8.36 ± 0.74 and 7.48 ± 0.27 mg/g, respectively) and phosphorylase a activities (2.32 ± 0.30 and 2.01 ± 0.43 μmoles released P_i/g/min, respectively) before coronary artery ligation were low compared with those obtained in saline-pretreated dogs. Pretreatment with carteolol also inhibited incompletely the changes in the glycogen level and phosphorylase a activity in both layers caused by coronary artery ligation. However, there were significant differences ($p < 0.01$) between the endocardial activity of phosphorylase a obtained before coronary artery ligation and that obtained after 1.5, 7, or 30 min of coronary artery ligation. After 30 min of coronary artery ligation, the epicardial phosphorylase a activity increased significantly ($p < 0.01$) and the endocardial glycogen level decreased significantly ($p < 0.01$).

Hexose Monophosphates and Beta Blockers
in Ischemic Myocardium

Figure 3 shows the changes in the levels of hexose monophosphates (G1P, G6P, and F6P) in the endo- and epicardial layers before and after coronary

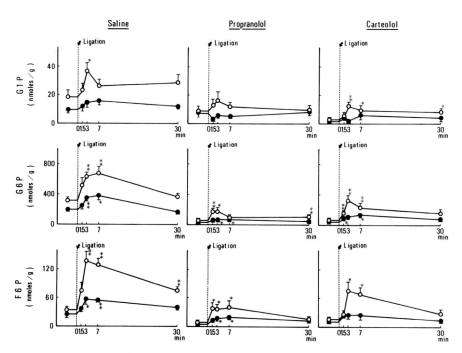

FIG. 3. Changes in endo- and epicardial G1P *(upper panel)*, G6P *(middle panel)*, and F6P *(lower panel)* after coronary artery ligation in the presence or absence of a beta-adrenergic blocker. (*Open circles,* endocardial layers; *solid circles,* epicardial layers.) For additional information, see Fig. 2.

artery ligation in the presence or absence of propranolol and carteolol. In saline-pretreated dogs, the endocardial levels of hexose monophosphates (G1P, G6P, and F6P: 0.018 ± 0.005, 0.313 ± 0.038, and 0.033 ± 0.007 μmoles/g, respectively) before coronary ligation were slightly higher than the epicardial levels (0.009 ± 0.002, 0.192 ± 0.020, and 0.024 ± 0.006 μmoles/g, respectively). All the hexose monophosphate levels in the endocardial layers increased rapidly and markedly after coronary artery ligation. The endocardial levels of G1P, G6P, and F6P after 3 min of coronary artery ligation were two, two, and four times, respectively, those obtained before coronary ligation. The epicardial hexose monophosphate levels, however, did not change as markedly as the endocardial. The increased hexose monophosphate levels in both layers tended to decrease within 30 min after coronary artery ligation.

In propranolol-pretreated dogs, the endo- and epicardial hexose monophosphate levels before coronary artery ligation were very low compared with saline-pretreated dogs. Pretreatment with propranolol almost prevented the changes in hexose monophosphate levels caused by coronary artery ligation. The levels of G6P and F6P in the endocardial layers, however, increased significantly after coronary artery ligation.

Carteolol injection also decreased markedly the levels of hexose monophosphates in both layers before coronary artery ligation. The increases in hexose monophosphate levels of both layers caused by coronary artery ligation were diminished by pretreatment with carteolol. Since the hexose monophosphate levels in both layers were low before coronary artery ligation in the presence of carteolol, the increases in these levels after coronary artery ligation were usually significant ($p < 0.05$ or $p < 0.01$), especially in the endocardial layers.

Pyruvate and Lactate Levels in Ischemic Myocardium in the Presence of Beta Blockers

Figure 4 shows changes in the pyruvate and lactate levels in the endo- and epicardial layers after coronary artery ligation in the presence or absence of a beta-adrenergic blocker.

In saline-pretreated dogs, the endocardial pyruvate (0.110 ± 0.023 μmoles/g) and lactate (3.20 ± 0.27 μmoles/g) levels were slightly higher than the epicardial (0.091 ± 0.014 and 2.44 ± 0.24 μmoles/g, respectively). Coronary artery ligation produced a slight change in the endo- and epicardial pyruvate levels, but the change was not significant. The lactate level increased rapidly and markedly after coronary artery ligation, especially in the endocardial layers. The increased levels of lactate in both layers caused by coronary artery ligation returned to the preligation levels 30 min after ligation.

In propranolol-pretreated dogs, the endo- and epicardial pyruvate (0.056 ± 0.008 and 0.046 ± 0.006 μmoles/g, respectively) and lactate (1.57 ± 0.21 and 1.36 ± 0.20 μmoles/g, respectively) levels before coronary ligation were lower

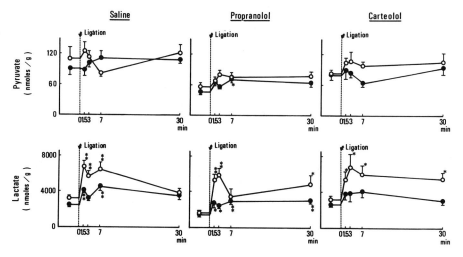

FIG. 4. Changes in endo- and epicardial pyruvate *(upper panel)* and lactate *(lower panel)* after coronary artery ligation in the presence or absence of a beta-adrenergic blocker. *(Open circles,* endocardial layers; *solid circles,* epicardial layers.) For additional information, see Fig. 2.

than those obtained in saline-pretreated dogs. After coronary artery ligation, there was a slight change in the endo- and epicardial pyruvate levels and a marked increase in the endocardial lactate level, as was seen in saline-pretreated dogs. The increase in the endocardial lactate level caused by coronary artery ligation, however, was transient.

In carteolol-pretreated dogs, the endo- and epicardial pyruvate (0.083 ± 0.003 and 0.082 ± 0.012 μmoles/g, respectively) and lactate levels (3.13 ± 0.35 and 2.60 ± 0.28 μmoles/g, respectively) did not significantly differ from those obtained in saline-pretreated dogs. Even in the presence of carteolol, coronary artery ligation produced a slight change in the endo- and epicardial pyruvate levels and a marked increase in the endocardial lactate level. These changes in the pyruvate and lactate levels caused by coronary artery ligation were similar to those obtained in saline-pretreated dogs.

Changes in Myocardial pH During Ischemia

A typical pattern of changes in regional pH of the myocardium measured by a glass pH microelectrode during and after ischemia is illustrated in Fig. 5. Immediately after a small branch of the coronary artery was ligated, the regional myocardial pH started to become markedly acidic (myocardial pH decrease). The myocardial pH, however, returned to the preligation level rapidly after release of the ligated coronary artery.

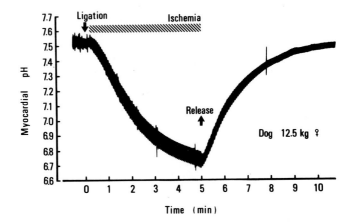

FIG. 5. A typical pattern of changes in myocardial pH before and after coronary artery ligation and after release of the ligation. Myocardial pH was continuously measured by a glass pH microelectrode inserted into the region of myocardium that was expected to become ischemic after coronary artery ligation. The small branch of the coronary artery was ligated and then released 5 min later.

Effect of Beta Blockers on Myocardial pH During Ischemia

Figure 6 shows the results obtained in two subgroups of pH experiments concerned with the effect of propranolol on changes in myocardial pH caused by coronary artery ligation and by isoproterenol injection.

In the first subgroup of experiments, regional pH in normal myocardium (before ligation) was 7.57 ± 0.07. Myocardial pH started to decrease immediately

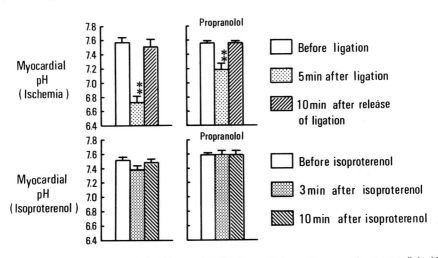

FIG. 6. Effects of pretreatment with propranolol (1 mg/kg) on decrease in myocardial pH caused by coronary artery ligation *(upper panel)* and by isoproterenol injection *(lower panel)*. Values are expressed as mean ± SE *(bars)*.

after coronary artery ligation and reached 6.73 ± 0.09 after 5 min of ligation. The difference between preligation and postligation levels of myocardial pH was significant ($p < 0.01$). After release of a 5-min ligation, myocardial pH increased rapidly to preligation levels. The myocardial pH 10 min after blood flow was restored was 7.51 ± 0.10. Pretreatment with propranolol attenuated the changes in myocardial pH caused by coronary artery ligation. In the presence of propranolol, the myocardial pH decreased to 7.20 ± 0.09 ($p < 0.01$) 5 min after coronary artery ligation and returned to the preligation level 10 min after release of coronary ligation.

In the other subgroup of experiments, regional myocardial pH decreased slightly from 7.51 ± 0.04 to 7.39 ± 0.06 3 min after isoproterenol injection, but the difference was not significant. The decreased pH, however, returned to the preinjection level within at least 10 min of isoproterenol injection. Pretreatment with propranolol prevented completely the change in myocardial pH caused by isoproterenol injection.

DISCUSSION

In the first group of experiments (metabolic experiment), it was found that coronary artery ligation accelerated breakdown of glycogen, elevated phosphorylase activity, and caused the accumulation of hexose monophosphates in the ischemic region, especially in the endocardial layers, and that pretreatment with the beta-adrenergic blocking drugs propranolol and carteolol (22) completely or partially inhibited these metabolic responses to ischemia (Figs. 2 and 3). It is well known that the oxygen deprivation produced by ischemia or anoxia causes acceleration of myocardial glycogenolysis and accumulation of the intermediates of glycolysis in the myocardium (8,11,16,18). However, the mechanisms of acceleration of myocardial metabolism during ischemia or anoxia are not fully understood.

Mayer (12) reported that pronethalol prevented the decrease in glycogen level in rat hearts caused by ischemia, but did not prevent the decrease in the glycogen level caused by anoxia. According to another report (4), practolol inhibits the increases in the cyclic adenosine 3',5'-monophosphate (cyclic AMP) level and in the phosphorylase activity after ischemia. In anoxic hearts, however, the change in the cyclic AMP level is inhibited by practolol, but the change in the phosphorylase activity is not. Mayer concluded from these findings that, although the response of myocardial glycogenolysis to ischemia and that to anoxia were similar, there was a difference between the mechanisms of the acceleration of glycogenolysis during ischemia and anoxia (12). Wollenberger (20) also reported that pronethalol prevented significant changes in the cyclic AMP level and phosphorylase activity during ischemia in dog hearts. These findings suggest that coronary artery ligation may produce the release of catecholamines or catecholamine-like substances which then accelerate glycogenolysis in the ischemic region supplied by the ligated coronary artery.

The levels of hexose monophosphates were decreased by propranolol or carteolol injection before coronary artery ligation, probably because the inflow of carbohydrates from glycogen to the glycolytic pathway decreases as a result of inhibition of glycogenolysis by propranolol or carteolol. Even in the presence of propranolol or carteolol, however, coronary artery ligation increased slightly and transiently the levels of hexose monophosphates. Neely (14) has demonstrated that reduction of coronary blood flow accelerates the rate of glucose utilization in isolated rat hearts. Therefore, it is likely that the hexose monophosphate levels would increase during coronary artery ligation even in the presence of beta blockers. Regardless of pretreatment with propranolol or carteolol, coronary artery ligation did not affect appreciably the endo- and epicardial pyruvate levels (Fig. 4). The lactate level, especially in the endocardial layers, increased immediately after coronary artery ligation, even in the presence of propranolol or carteolol. It is difficult to explain why propranolol or carteolol did not modify the changes in lactate level after coronary artery ligation, despite the fact that these drugs inhibit the acceleration of glycogenolysis and the accumulation of hexose monophosphates after ischemia. It is possible to assume, however, that the increase in lactate resulted from the inhibition of flow from the glycolytic pathway to the tricarboxylic acid cycle (TCA cycle) and the acceleration of glucose utilization caused by ischemia.

Before discussing the results obtained in the second group of experiments (pH experiment), it should be mentioned that the method for determination of myocardial pH using a glass pH microelectrode inserted into the myocardium does not measure intracellular or extracellular pH; rather, it measures the pH of a mixture containing intra- and extracellular fluid. It is assumed, however, that the pH reflects intracellular pH, because alteration in the intracellular pH influences the extracellular pH (14,16).

When the oxygen supply to myocardial cells decreases, the myocardial pH decreases (Fig. 5). There is considerable evidence to support this phenomenon. Results obtained by determination of myocardial pH according to the method using 5,5-dimethyloxazolidine-2,4-dion (DMO) (14), pH indicator paper (10), or pH electrode (6) indicate that myocardial pH decreases during ischemia. Why does myocardial pH decrease during ischemia? Recently, Gevers (7) described in detail how hydrogen ions could be generated by various processes of metabolism in heart cells and that acceleration of the metabolism during ischemia would increase the generation of hydrogen ions in the cardiac tissue. These hydrogen ions would accumulate in the ischemic region of the myocardium because of lack of blood flow. Since the accumulated hydrogen ions would be washed out after release of coronary artery ligation, the decreased myocardial pH would increase rapidly after the release of ligation.

Myocardial pH also decreased after isoproterenol injection. The decrease in myocardial pH after isoproterenol injection, however, was insignificant and transient. Propranolol pretreatment did not inhibit completely the decrease in myocardial pH caused by coronary artery ligation, although it inhibited completely the decrease in myocardial pH caused by isoproterenol injection. These findings suggest that beta-adrenergic receptors are partially involved in the mechanism of the decrease in myocardial pH caused by coronary artery ligation.

It is concluded that stimulation of beta-adrenergic receptors may be involved in the mechanisms of acceleration of glycogenolysis, accumulation of hexose monophosphates, and decrease of tissue pH in ischemic myocardial region. However, whether catecholamines are directly or only indirectly involved in changes in myocardial metabolism during ischemia remains to be clarified.

ACKNOWLEDGMENT

The authors thank Mr. T. Yokoyama for his valuable technical assistance.

REFERENCES

1. Barker, S. B., and Summerson, W. H. (1941): The colorimetric determination of lactic acid in biological material. *J. Biol. Chem.*, 138:535–554.
2. Bergmeyer, H.-U., editor (1974): *Methods of Enzymatic Analysis,* pp. 1233–1242 (G1P, G6P, and F6P), pp. 1446–1448 (pyruvate). Academic Press, New York.
3. Bing, R. J. (1965): Cardiac metabolism. *Physiol. Rev.,* 45:171–213.
4. Dobson, J. G., Jr., and Mayer, S. E. (1973): Mechanisms of activation of cardiac glycogen phosphorylase in ischemia and anoxia. *Circ. Res.,* 33:412–420.
5. Fiske, C. H., and Subbarow, Y. (1925): The colorimetric determination of phosphorus. *J. Biol. Chem.,* 66:375–400.
6. Gebert, G., Benzing, H., and Strohm, M. (1971): Changes in interstitial pH of dog myocardium in response to local ischemia, hypoxia, hyper- and hypocapnia, measured continuously by means of glass microelectrodes. *Pfluegers Arch.,* 329:72–81.
7. Gevers, W. (1977): Generation of protons by metabolic processes in heart cells. *J. Mol. Cell. Cardiol.,* 9:867–874.
8. Ichihara, K., and Abiko, Y. (1975): Difference between endocardial and epicardial utilization of glycogen in the ischemic heart. *Am. J. Physiol.,* 229:1585–1589.
9. Ichihara, K., and Abiko, Y. (1977): Crossover-plot analysis of glycolytic intermediates in canine ischemic myocardium after coronary artery ligation. *Jpn. J. Pharmacol. (Suppl.),* 27:99.
10. Krug, A. (1975): Alterations in myocardial hydrogen ion concentration after temporary coronary occlusion: A sign of irreversible cell damage. *Am. J. Cardiol.,* 36:214–217.
11. Kübler, W., and Spieckermann, P. G. (1970): Regulation of glycolysis in the ischemic and the anoxic myocardium. *J. Mol. Cell. Cardiol.,* 1:351–377.
12. Mayer, S. E. (1974): Effect of catecholamines on cardiac metabolism. *Circ. Res. (Suppl. III),* 34, 35:III-129–III-137.
13. Neely, J. R., Rovetto, M. J., and Oram, J. F. (1972): Myocardial utilization of carbohydrate and lipids. *Prog. Cardiovasc. Dis.,* 15:289–329.
14. Neely, J. R., Whitmer, J. T., and Rovetto, M. J. (1975): Effect of coronary blood flow of glycolytic flux and intracellular pH in isolated rat hearts. *Circ. Res.,* 37:733–741.
15. Opie, L. H. (1968): Metabolism of the heart in health and disease. Part I. *Am. Heart J.,* 76:685–698.
16. Opie, L. H. (1976): Effects of regional ischemia on metabolism of glucose and fatty acids. Relative rates of aerobic and anaerobic energy production during myocardial infarction and comparison with effects of anoxia. *Circ. Res. (Suppl. I),* 38:I-52–I-74.
17. Seifter, S., Dayton, S., Novic, B., and Muntwyler, E. (1950): The estimation of glycogen with the anthrone reagent. *Arch. Biochem. Biophys.,* 25:191–200.
18. Wollenberger, A., and Krause, E.-G. (1963): Activation of α-glucan phosphorylase and related metabolic changes in dog myocardium. *Biochim. Biophys. Acta,* 67:337–340.
19. Wollenberger, A., and Krause, E.-G. (1968): Metabolic control characteristics of the acutely ischemic myocardium. *Am. J. Cardiol.,* 22:349–359.

20. Wollenberger, A., Krause, E.-G., and Heier, G. (1969): Stimulation of 3′,5′-cyclic AMP formation in dog myocardium following arrest of blood flow. *Biochem. Biophys. Res. Commun.,* 36:664–670.
21. Wollenberger, A., and Shahab, L. (1965): Anoxia-induced release of noradrenaline from the isolated perfused heart. *Nature,* 207:88–89.
22. Yabuuchi, Y., and Kinoshita, D. (1974): Cardiovascular studies of 5-(3-tert-butylamino-2-hydroxy) propoxy-3,4-dihydrocarbostyril hydrochloride (OPC-1085), a new potent β-adrenergic blocking agent. *Jpn. J. Pharmacol.,* 24:853–861.

Ischemic Myocardium and Antianginal Drugs,
edited by M. M. Winbury and Y. Abiko.
Raven Press, New York © 1979.

Altered Permeability and Volume Elasticity During Transient Ischemia

Tomiyasu Koyama, Yuji Kikuchi, and Yoshihiro Kakiuchi

Research Institute of Applied Electricity, Hokkaido University, Sapporo 060, Japan

According to the Starling mechanism (15), water moves into the interstitial space at the arteriolar end of the capillary and back into the capillary at the venular end as a consequence of the interaction of hydraulic and osmotic forces. The amount of water that moves across the capillary walls is enormous. An amount equal to the entire plasma volume enters and leaves the tissues in one day (10). Such a water turnover occurs in the myocardium to transport products of the metabolic chemical chains and to facilitate movements of large molecules. Once the blood flow is interrupted, not only is the fluid circulation (i.e., waste transport mechanisms), but also the steady turnover of the chemical reactions probably disturbed. Presently, however, we have relatively little knowledge of what happens in the water circulation in tissues.

The movement of water from the tissues into the capillary blood, i.e., absorption, was confirmed by the weight loss of isolated and perfused organs including hearts by a step increase in the colloid osmotic pressure of the perfusate (2,17). However, with respect to these measurements, the following questions arise: Was the fluid content of these tissues actually at the same level as the *in vivo* fluid content? And can absorption occur in the more physiological states (6)? Meanwhile, only the filtration process was confirmed by the micropipette and microocclusion technique in the mesentery and omentum (6). Since the reverse movement of water back from the tissue into the capillary—i.e., absorption—could hardly be observed, the circulation of water in tissues themselves is doubted (6).

In this chapter, the available publications on myocardial water movement are briefly surveyed, and changes in water balance are analyzed in the myocardium exposed to ischemia.

WEIGHT TRANSIENT METHOD

Water movements across the capillary wall were often studied by means of the weight transient method. Isolated rabbit hearts were continuously weighed while both the arterial and venous pressures were adjusted so as to maintain the weights at constant levels (17). Each heart was initially perfused with Ringer's solution containing no test molecules. Then a sudden switch was made to Ringer's solution containing a small amount of one of the test substances. Since each substance was osmotically active, the heart lost weight as a function of time. The initial transcapillary flow was 2.1×10^{-2} g/sec and 7.5×10^{-2} g/sec in the whole heart when sucrose, 10 and 50 mM, respectively, was added to the perfusate (17). Since 1 mOsmole of solute corresponds to 17 mm Hg of osmotic pressure, these doses elevated colloid osmotic pressure (COP) of the perfusate by 170 and 850 mm Hg. Initially after sucrose was added, these osmotic pressures acted to absorb water from tissues into capillaries. Rough calculations from the data yielded values of the water filtration coefficient of the order of 10^{-11} cm/(sec·dyn·cm^{-2}). Semilogarithmic plots of the weight losses formed linear and parallel curves over a time period of 25 sec. This relation was interpreted to indicate an asymptotic increase of the extravascular concentration of the solute. Moreover, it was concluded that the passive transport of solvent across the capillary walls related to the hydrostatic pressure difference and solute concentration differences existing across the capillary blood and extravascular spaces.

Interpretation of such data, however, requires realistic mathematical modeling in order to yield valid estimates of permeability (2). These phenomena include permeation of the capillary membrane by native and test solutes; water permeation across parenchymal cell membranes; tissue-dependent volumes of distribution for solutes in the interstitium; time-dependent cell, interstitial, and capillary hydrostatic pressures; solute buffering of water movements by impermeable solutes and the native electrolyte; and possible partial flow limitation to transcapillary exchange. For osmotic weight transients, one must additionally account for transcapillary water flow in response to osmotic and hydrostatic pressure gradients and solvent drag. Grabowski (2) took all these effects into account in a multisolute model for osmotic weight transients of myocardium. Transcapillary fluxes of solutes and the solvent are given by multisolute Kedem–Katchalsky relations. Complicated numerical calculations of the model lead to interdependent estimates of coefficients for capillary filtration, permeability, and reflection that are strongly affected by solute buffering and changes in tissue hydrostatic pressure. Myocardial tissue stiffness and water permeability of the myocardial cell membrane constitute nonnegligible contributions to the weight transient.

In spite of these efforts, there remain questions inherent in the weight transient method as pointed out by Intaglietta (6): Is the amount of free water *in vivo* and *in situ* comparable to that under particular experimental conditions? And do the water movements observed under the experimental conditions actually occur in the living animals? Apart from myocardial tissues, Intaglietta and Zweifach (7) found that in the mesentery of various animals, more than 85% of the capillaries tested showed outward motion of fluid (i.e., filtration). In 15% of the capillaries studied by the microocclusion technique, red blood cells remained stationary after occlusion except in a few instances in which their motion could be attributed to absorption. Also in rat cremaster muscle, Smaje et al.

(14) noted that filtration was predominant through the capillary network of this tissue. Absorption was found to occur in small venules of the order of 12 μm in diameter, where macromolecules can move across the vascular wall; therefore, colloid osmotic pressure could not affect the fluid movements.

Comprehensive surveys of the distribution of microvascular pressure by means of the resistance servo nulling technique have become available (18). Intaglietta (6) reported that the capillary hydraulic pressure (except in the venular capillaries) was found to be consistently higher than the colloid osmotic pressure measured by membrane osmometer. It is apparent that the Starling concept of fluid balance is not fulfilled in the conditions tested. Thus, it seems necessary to approach the extravascular fluid circulation by means of a different method.

CONTINUOUS MEASUREMENTS OF COLLOID OSMOTIC PRESSURE DURING REACTIVE HYPEREMIA

We were interested in experimental procedures that were less artificial than the perfusion of isolated hearts and step changes in colloid osmotic pressure. As one such procedure, we tested continuous measurements of colloid osmotic pressure and observed the effects of reactive hyperemia on water movements between capillary blood and myocardium (8). It was assumed that the colloid osmotically active substance in the blood was protein, since the concentrations of the other macromolecular substances were relatively low and, therefore, that changes in colloid osmotic pressure in the blood were mainly attributable to changes in protein concentration resulting from water filtration or absorption. In other words, it was expected that changes in the amount of water in capillary blood were detectable as changes in colloid osmotic pressure.

Mongrel dogs were anesthetized with pentobarbital. Ventilation was maintained by a positive pressure respirator. The heart was exposed by a thoracotomy made at the fourth intercostal space. The anterior descending branch of the left coronary artery (LAD) was threaded with a thin suture for coronary arterial occlusion. A soft polyethylene tube (2.0 mm o.d., 1.4 mm i.d., and 30 cm long) was introduced into the great cardiac vein via the left jugular vein. The proximal end of this tube was connected to a plastic tube that was fixed to a double peristaltic pump. The proximal end of the plastic tube was connected to the colloid osmometer (13). After heparinization of the dog, the peristaltic pump was turned on and adjusted to pump blood at the rate of 4.0 ml/min. Thus, the cardiac venous blood flowed through the colloid osmometer, allowing continuous measurement of colloid osmotic pressure. The blood sample returned into the right femoral vein through another plastic tube fixed to the double peristaltic pump. The colloid osmometer was calibrated with albumin–water solutions with osmotic pressures which had been determined by means of a freezing point depression osmometer. Since the colloid osmotic pressure rose steadily because of the thoracotomy, saline was continuously infused into the left femoral vein at the rate of 5.0 ml/min. Aortic blood pressure was recorded

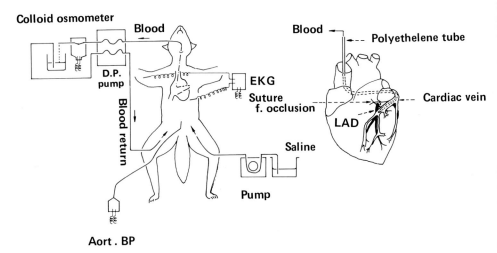

FIG. 1. Schematic illustration of experimental set-up. LAD, anterior descending branch of left coronary artery; DP pump, double peristaltic pump used for continuous sampling and infusion of cardiac venous blood; Aort. BP, aortic blood pressure. (From Koyama et al., ref. 9, with permission).

via a polyethylene tube placed in the descending aorta. The complete experimental setup is shown in Fig. 1.

A sample recording is shown in Fig. 2. The curves from top to bottom represent aortic blood pressure (aortic BP) and colloid osmotic pressure (COP) with low and high magnifications (COP 1 and 2, respectively). The recordings were transiently interrupted at points indicated by open arrows. The thick horizontal bars indicated the time period of the LAD occlusion (30, 60, 120, and 240 sec). From 30 to 90 sec after the occlusion was released, COP rose and then fell transiently; after 90 sec, it became lower than the initial level and recovered gradually. The period during which COP was lower than the initial level became longer as occlusion time was prolonged. The right side of the recording shows where the colloid osmometer system was switched to draw saline instead of cardiac venous blood. The COP 1 curve quickly fell and showed an overshoot, reaching a plateau within 90 sec, while the COP 2 curve went off the scale. An electronic signal that corresponded to 20 mm Hg of COP was recorded for calibration. Then the system was again switched to cardiac venous blood. The COP 1 curve quickly rose and returned to the initial level after an overshoot. During this series of measurements, the peristaltic pump continued to draw blood from the great cardiac vein.

In another series of measurements, the peristaltic pump was stopped during the LAD occlusion. In this case, the COP signal rose slightly during the pump arrest because red blood cells in the osmometer were deposited on the membrane (5). But when the drawing action of the pump was restored, the COP signal returned quickly to the initial level and then showed a sharp rise followed by a slower transient decrease below the preocclusion level.

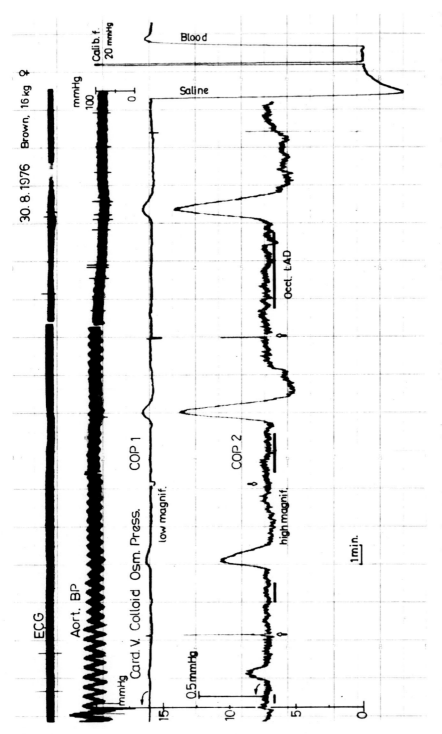

FIG. 2. Typical experimental recording. Curves from top to bottom: aortic blood pressure, colloid osmotic pressure of cardiac venous blood recorded with low (COP 1) and high (COP 2) magnification. *Horizontal bars* below COP 2 tracing indicate the LAD occlusion period. *Open arrows* indicate transient interruption of recording. (From Koyama et al., ref. 9, with permission).

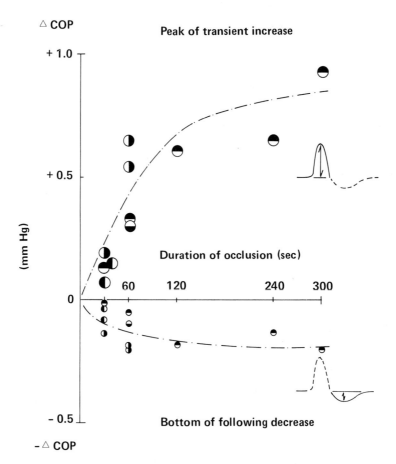

FIG. 3. Relationship between COP changes and duration of LAD occlusion. Peak of COP increase (Δ COP, *top curve*) and bottom of decrease (−Δ COP, *bottom curve*), shown schematically with arrows in the top and bottom insets, are plotted on the ordinate. Since repetition and prolongation of coronary occlusion readily caused arrhythmia, occlusion tests were made only a few times in each case. (From Koyama et al., ref. 9, with permission).

The amplitudes of COP changes—the amplitudes of both the sharp increase (ΔCOP) and the following decrease below the initial level (−ΔCOP) as a function of occlusion time—are summarized for four dogs in Fig. 3. A saturation curve seems to relate COP and occlusion time (upper curve in Fig. 3). The rate of increase in ΔCOP was reduced when occlusion times were longer than 3 min. When occlusion times were longer than about 2 min, −ΔCOP remained almost constant (lower curve in Fig. 3).

The initial increase and the following gradual decrease in COP is interpreted as follows. During postocclusive reactive hyperemia, the arterioles were fully dilated. The capillary pressure rose, and water moved from the plasma into the tissue. The saturation curve (Fig. 3, upper curve) suggests a limitation of the water absorption capacity of myocardial tissue. As hyperemia ceased, capillary pressure decreased, and the excess amount of water that had been absorbed by the tissue flowed back slowly into the capillary blood. When the sample for COP measurements was changed from blood to saline, the COP signal showed an overshoot. This was caused only by a large change in the quality of the sample fluid. No such overshoot appeared in the COP signal when an albumin solution was added to the sample blood flowing through the osmometer. Therefore, no error due to the overshoot was included in the COP recording of cardiac venous blood.

ANALYSIS OF COP CHANGES

In the COP measurements it seems probable that water was filtered from the capillary blood and absorbed back into the blood from tissues, at least during and after reactive hyperemia, where the perfusion pressure changed greatly. In this case, water probably moves according to the hydrostatic pressure difference across capillary walls. We tried to see if these changes could successfully be analyzed on the basis of the Starling hypothesis.

Formulation of the Problem

Water flows from the plasma of the capillary blood into the interstitial tissue space and vice versa according to the pressure gradient existing between the plasma and the tissue (15). This relation is expressed in an analogy of Oka's and Murata's expression (11) by the following equation:

$$M = k \cdot (P - \alpha), \qquad [1]$$

and

$$\alpha = P_t + \Pi_p - \Pi_t, \qquad [2]$$

where M represents the rate of water movements; k the filtration coefficient; P and P_t the blood and tissue hydraulic pressures, respectively; and Π_p and Π_t, the plasma and tissue COPs, respectively. The term α is the sum of all the pressures that may act to cause water movement, except blood hydraulic pressure. Since Π_t is relatively small in actual tissues, α represents mainly the total value of P_t and Π_p, both opposing water filtration. Their effects can not be measured separately and both change theoretically in accordance with the amount of water moving from the blood into tissue.

A steady state solution of Navier–Stokes equation was employed in the preceding study to analyze COP changes (9). But an electronic analog model for a Krogh tissue cylinder shown in Fig. 4A seems to be more convenient for the analysis because fluid movements across capillary wall and through the tissue can easily be taken into consideration. The three factors contained in α can be introduced separately in an electronic model. However, the comprehensive term α was utilized for the ease of understanding. Blood flows at a rate of I_c

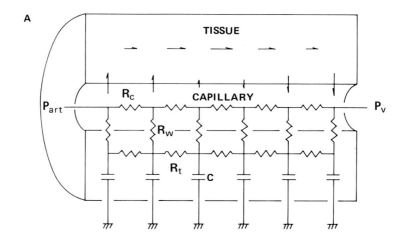

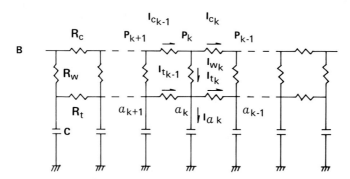

FIG. 4. A: A Krogh tissue cylinder showing corresponding resistances and capacitances. R_c, resistance for blood flow in capillary; R_w, resistance for water flow across capillary wall; R_t, resistance for water flow in tissue; C, interstitial space compliance. *Arrows* indicate directions of water movement. **B:** Analog model for blood and water flow in the tissue cylinder. P, hydraulic pressure in capillary; α, algebraic sum of tissue hydraulic pressure and plasma and tissue fluid colloid osmotic pressure; I_c, blood flow rate in capillary; I_w, water flow rate across capillary wall; I_t, water flow rate in tissue; I_a, rate of water accumulation in tissue; p, a point in the model circuit.

through the capillary having the resistance R_c according to the capillary pressure difference ΔP, which corresponds to the voltage difference applied to the resistance. A part of the fluid contained in the blood is filtered across the capillary wall having a resistance R_w at a rate of I_w into the tissue cylinder according to the pressure gradient between the pressure inside the capillary and that in the tissue cylinder $(P - \alpha)$. The filtered fluid flows at a rate of I_t through the tissue by the gradient of α against the resistance of R_t. These three factors can be represented with three electronic resistances. Furthermore, the fluid accumulates in the tissue and causes a repulsion against the further fluid inflow into the tissue, which can be expressed by a charging current for a capacitance C. The voltage applied to C corresponds to α, while the rate of water accumulation is the charging current I_a. P, α, I_c, I_w, I_t, and I_a are all different at each portion of the tissue cylinder. If the capillary is divided into several sections having a length of Δx, these properties can be expressed as a serial connection of several unit networks, as shown in Fig. 4B. Calculations on this model are described in the Appendix (Eqs. A1 to A16). Finally, we assume that mean capillary pressure P_{av} is expressed as the mean of capillary pressures at the arterial end (P_{art}) and venous end (P_v), which change with time according to the equation

$$P_{av} = \frac{1}{L}\int_0^L P\,dx = \frac{P_{art} + P_v}{2}.$$ [3]

Then the average of α (i.e., α_{av}) is given from Eq. A16 by the following equation:

$$\alpha_{av} = \frac{1}{R_w \cdot C} e^{-t/R_w} \cdot C \int_0^t e^{\tau/R_w \cdot C} \cdot P_{av}(\tau)d\tau + e^{-t/R_w \cdot C} \cdot \alpha_{av}|_{t=0}.$$ [4]

Since the rate of water movement (M) across the capillary walls is the sum of Q_w along the capillary length (see Appendix, Eq. A3), the following equation can be obtained:

$$M = \int_0^L I_w\,dx = \frac{1}{R_w}\int_0^L (P - \alpha)\,dx = \frac{1}{R_w}(P_{av} - \alpha_{av}).$$ [5]

Since changes in plasma COP—i.e., $\Delta\Pi/\Pi_p$ (hereafter abbreviated as $\Delta\Pi/\Pi$)—in venous blood are proportional to those in protein concentration, the following relation can be obtained (9):

$$\frac{\Delta\Pi}{\Pi} = \frac{M}{I_c(0) - M}$$ [6]

where $I_c(0)$ represents the blood flow at the arterial end of the capillary given by the Poiseuille equation.

Resistances and capacitance in these equations relate with the corresponding conductivities k_w and k_t and with the volume elasticity K by the following equations, respectively:

$$1/R_w = 2\pi \cdot b \cdot k_w$$
$$1/R_t = k_t \cdot \pi \cdot (d^2 - b^2)$$ [7]
$$1/C = K/[\pi \cdot (d^2 - b^2)]$$

where b and d represent radii of the capillary and tissue cylinder, respectively. Thus, $\Delta\Pi/\Pi$ is readily calculated by Eqs. 3 to 7, when P_{art} and P_v are measured.

Wedge Pressure Substituted for P_{art}

P_{art} and P_v should be measured directly by a method such as the micropipette technique. But it seemed impossible to use this technique for strongly beating hearts. Instead, we measured the wedge pressure P_{wedge} with a catheter introduced via the jugular vein and tightly wedged in a fine branch of the cardiac vein, in an analogy of the routine measurement of pulmonary capillary and pulmonary venous pressures by means of a catheter wedged in a branch of the pulmonary artery. We assumed that P_{wedge} could represent the perfusion pressure for the myocardial capillary network. When a small branch of cardiac vein is stopped by the tip of a catheter, the local network of microvasculature may be exposed to a partial congestion and the pressure there may be slightly increased. However, since local myocardial vasculatures are connected with those in the other portions through arteriolar anastomoses (1), the pressure will equilibrate with the perfusion pressure acting on the arterial end of the capillary network of the intact portions. Although the pattern of the transmitted pressure may partly be modified by the compression of myocardium, P_{wedge} seems to represent the perfusion pressure better than the LAD pressure does; the systolic pressure of P_{wedge} is only 60 mm Hg during the normal perfusion and is increased by reactive hyperemia. A peripheral cardiac venous pressure was recorded as P_v with a catheter whose tip was slightly withdrawn from the wedge position. The mean values of P_{wedge} and P_v are traced together in Fig. 5. P_{wedge} is usually higher than P_v and decreases more quickly than P_v when the LAD is occluded. After release of LAD occlusion, P_{wedge} increases rapidly and transiently attains much higher values than during the control condition. Meanwhile, P_v follows slower time courses.

Calculated Time Courses in COP and α During Hyperemia

The time courses of $\Delta\Pi/\Pi$ and α were calculated by putting the mean P_{wedge} and P_v into the above equations. The size of the tissue cylinder was assumed: $b = 3$ μm, $d = 14$ μm, and L (length) $= 1$ mm (16). When suitable values of k_w and K are selected, the time courses of the obtained $\Delta\Pi/\Pi$ agreed with the actually recorded COP patterns with 10% for both the amount of COP increase and the duration. Such an example for 2-min LAD occlusion is shown in Fig. 6 (top). COP increased sharply after the release of occlusion, then decreased below the preocclusion level and gradually recovered. The time course of α shown in Fig. 6 (bottom) suggests the factors contributing to such COP changes. The value of α, which mainly acts to oppose water filtration, rose rather slowly and attained the maximum value when the COP curve crossed the zero line. The force counteracting the water filtration was elevated by the increment in perfusion pressure with a time lag, so as to attain the maximum value in proportion to the amount of filtered water. Then it decreased slowly to the normal level, causing the COP level to fall below the control level for

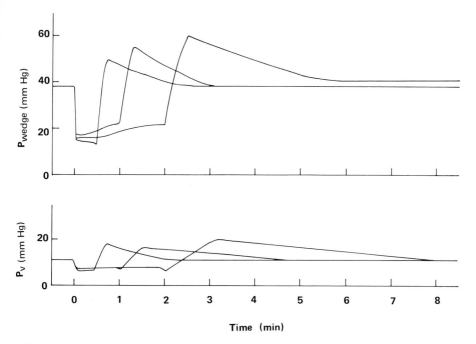

FIG. 5. Time courses of mean wedge pressure (P_{wedge}) and peripheral cardiac venous pressure (P_v) are traced for three occlusion periods.

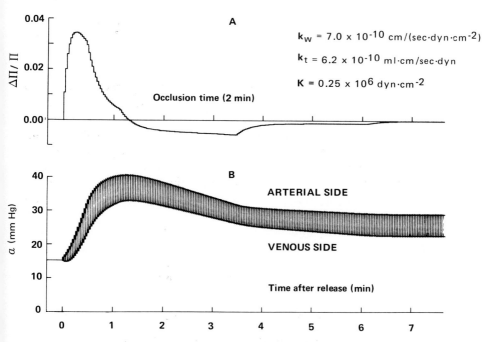

$k_w = 7.0 \times 10^{-10}$ cm/(sec·dyn·cm^{-2})

$k_t = 6.2 \times 10^{-10}$ ml·cm/sec·dyn

$K = 0.25 \times 10^6$ dyn·cm^{-2}

Occlusion time (2 min)

ARTERIAL SIDE

VENOUS SIDE

Time after release (min)

FIG. 6. Example of time course of changes in plasma colloid osmotic pressure $(\Delta \Pi / \Pi)$ **(A)** and α **(B)** calculated for 2 min LAD occlusion. Output from the calculator was directly recorded on an x–y recorder.

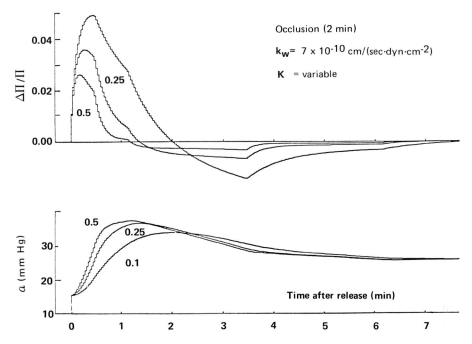

FIG. 7. Effects of K value on the calculated α *(t)* and $\Delta\Pi/\Pi$ values. The value for k_w used for calculations was kept constant: 7.0×10^{-10} cm/(sec·dyn·cm^{-2}). See text for definitions of variables. (From Koyama et al., ref. 9, with permission.)

a few minutes. One of the main components of α is the hydraulic pressure in the myocardial tissue space, which may have proper stiffness or volume elasticity. The contribution of stiffness or volume elasticity to water filtration was discussed by Grabowski and Bassingthwaighte (2) and Koyama et al. (8). Although this contribution has not been discussed seriously in most weight transient measurements, its importance for controlling water filtration can clearly be seen in Fig. 7. Time courses of COP are calculated for the same k_w, P_{wedge}, and P_v, using several arbitrarily chosen K values. If K is small or zero, COP remains increased for too long a time period, while changes in COP calculated using large K values are too small and of short duration. The adequately sharp and transient changes appear only with a suitable K value. In a similar manner, the effects of a certain K value on COP are greatly affected by k_w values. Thus, the ranges of acceptable k_w and K values are unexpectedly limited.

Quick Changes in k_w and K Values

Specific combinations of k_w and K values are required to obtain an agreement between the calculated and experimentally recorded COP curves for each occlusion time. In Fig. 8, these values obtained in serial measurements are plotted

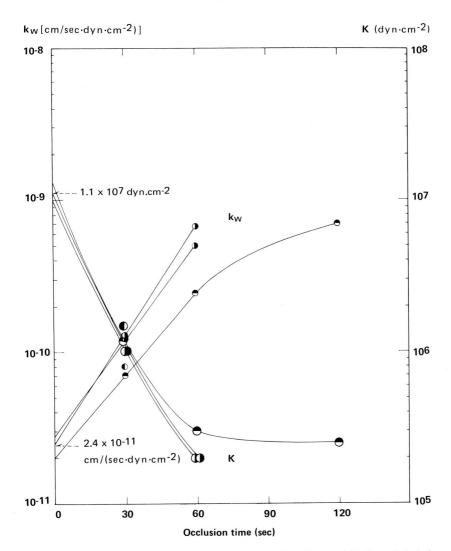

FIG. 8. Relation between the duration of LAD occlusion and k_w values and K values. Calculations of $\Delta \Pi / \Pi$, using suitable k_w and K values, yielded time courses coinciding with the actually recorded COP curves. The suitable k_w and K values changed with different durations of LAD occlusion. (From Koyama et al., ref. 9, with permission.)

against the occlusion time. The water permeability k_w increases, while the myocardial volume elasticity K decreases quickly with the prolongation of LAD occlusion. The values for k_w and K under normal conditions estimated by extrapolation of the curves to the abscissa are 2.4×10^{-11} cm/(sec·dyn·cm^{-2}) and 1.1×10^{7} dyn·cm^{-2}, respectively.

This result indicates that drastic changes occur rapidly in water permeability of the capillary wall and volume elasticity of the interstitial space. According to Powell et al. (12), a transient period of regional myocardial ischemia results in morphologic changes which include myocardial and capillary endothelial cell swelling. The administration of hyperosmotic mannitol reduces the amount of ischemic cell swelling, which presumably improves collateral blood flow to the ischemic area. This salutary effect may be a common property of hyperosmolar agents. Thus, Powell et al. (22) emphasized the importance of diminishing the cell swelling. Figure 8 indicates that factors involved in the system for extravascular circulation change parallel to or prior to morphological changes of myocardial cells. The changes permit filtration of more water into the interstitial space and presumably contribute to the acceleration of cell swelling.

The data on COP and pressures used for the present estimation of k_w and K values were obtained in separate measurements, and the theoretical analysis requires several assumptions. The dead space of the measuring system causes a time lag before the system responds to COP changes. The slow flow rate in the catheter may average out the changes in recorded osmotic pressure. The response of the membrane osmometer was 60% in 15 sec. This slow response may cause some modification in the COP recording. Therefore, it can only be expected to clarify the relative changes in k_w and K values. In spite of these technical difficulties, the estimated k_w value under the control condition was similar to the value reported for the muscle capillary (10) and was in the same order as the roughly estimated value from Vargas and Johnson's result in rabbit heart (17).

Guyton (3) has determined the pressure–volume curve of the interstitial space in the isolated hind limb of the dog and has obtained a compliance of 0.4 ml/mm Hg·100 g tissue, which can be converted to 2.7×10^6 dyn·cm^{-2} as the volume elasticity. The K value under normal conditions obtained in the present study is slightly greater than that of Guyton. This difference, however, seems reasonable considering the powerful contraction of the myocardium and the assumptions required for the calculation of the K value.

Thus, the water movement during and after reactive hyperemia can be explained mostly by the Starling hypothesis combined with the volume elasticity of the interstitial space. Reactive hyperemia may be a case where a substantial amount of fluid is filtered into the interstitial space and there is a balance between filtration and absorption, as stated by Intaglietta (6).

Flow Rate in the Extravascular Circulation in Steady State

For the calculation of the curves in Fig. 6, the minimum value reported for the abdominal subcutaneous tissues by Guyton et al. (4) was tentatively used for k_t. Although the k_t value had no essential effect on the time courses of COP, it is seen that α is higher on the arterial side than on the venous side of the capillary. The contribution of the k_t value to water movement in tissue will be clear when steady state water balance is discussed.

Steady state solution of Eqs. A11 and A12 gives P and α by the following equations:

$$P = Be^{\gamma x} + De^{-\gamma x} - \frac{1}{\gamma^2}(bx + d), \qquad [8]$$

$$\alpha = \frac{R_t}{R_c}(Be^{\gamma x} + De^{-\gamma x}) - \frac{1}{\gamma^2}(bx + d), \qquad [9]$$

where

$$\gamma^2 = \frac{R_c + R_t}{R_w},$$

$$B = (P_{art} - P_v) / \left[2(1 - e^{\gamma L}) - \frac{L \cdot R_t \cdot \gamma}{R_c} \cdot \frac{e^{\gamma L} - e^{-\gamma L}}{1 - e^{-\gamma L}} \right],$$

$$D = \frac{1 - e^{\gamma L}}{1 - e^{-\gamma L}} \cdot B, \qquad [10]$$

$$b = -\frac{R_t \cdot \gamma^3}{R_c}(B - D),$$

$$d = \gamma^2 \cdot (B + D - P_{art}).$$

Now, the values for k_t as well as k_w are required to calculate P and α from eqs. 8 and 9. The data on the hydraulic permeability of tissue were first obtained by Guyton et al. (4) from measurements on the rate of fluid transfer between two capsules implanted in the subcutaneous tissue of the dog. The value reported was 18×10^{-10} ml·cm/sec·dyn. A lower value of the order of 0.45×10^{-10} ml·cm/sec·dyn can be deduced from the data reported by Winter and Kruger (19). Recent measurements in the laboratory of Intaglietta (6) on the hydraulic conductivity of mesenteric membranes gave a value of the order of 2×10^{-10} ml·cm/sec·dyn.

Assuming k_w and k_t to be 6.1×10^{-10} ml·cm/sec·dyn and 2.0×10^{-10} ml·cm/sec·dyn, respectively, for the mesentery, we calculated the values for P and α along a tissue cylinder and plotted them in Fig. 9. A clear gradient in α appeared along the longitudinal axis. Unfortunately, we had no information on myocardial k_t. As an order estimation, we sought a k_t value that yielded the same P and α patterns as those of the mesentery. We repeated the calculation using the k_w obtained in the myocardium and arbitrarily chosen k_t values, so that we could finally obtain the same patterns. The k_t value for normal conditions was 7.7×10^{-12} ml·cm/sec·dyn. If the same relation between P and α could be maintained even for increased k_w, k_t values would increase remarkably. The triangular area enclosed by the P and α curves multiplied by the capillary wall permeability k_w yields the total flow rate of extravascular circulation in tissue. The relationship between the total flow rate and k_t can be obtained with k_w as a parameter. Such an example is shown in Fig. 10. Four k_w values, three obtained for the three occlusion periods and one for the normal condition, were employed. Estimated k_t values are denoted with arrows on the correspond-

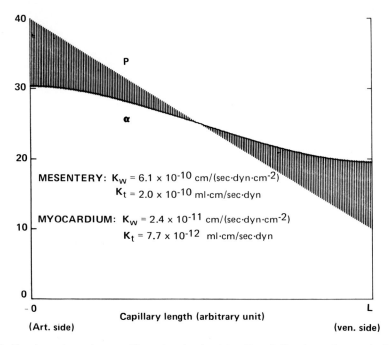

FIG. 9. P and α values along capillary at a steady state. P_a and P_v values of preocclusion in Fig. 7 are used for the calculation.

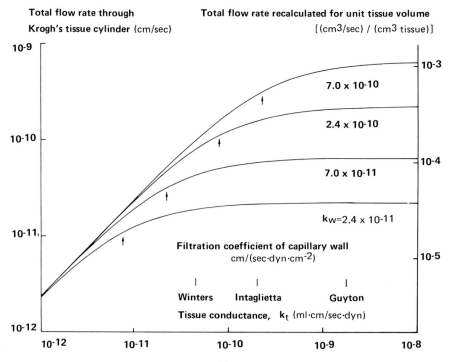

FIG. 10. Relation between total flow rate in tissue and tissue conductance for water flow (k_t) with a parameter of water permeability of capillary wall (k_w).

ing curves. At the extreme case where $k_t = 0$, the tissue cylinder is not perfused. When k_t is sufficiently large, the total flow rate in tissue simply depends on k_w. In the range between these extreme cases, total flow rate is restricted by a combination of k_w and k_t. The available k_t values published by the three authors previously mentioned are indicated by vertical lines in the lower part of the figure. They distribute in the k_t range where the relations are curving. Although the present estimations contain much uncertainty, the range of estimated k_t values overlaps the range of the published data. In addition, the extravascular circulation probably increases when exposed to ischemia. The total flow rate in tissue during normal conditions is estimated to be smaller than 0.1% of the total capillary flow, which may flow to the lymphatic capillaries, as mentioned by Intaglietta. Total flow rate in tissue increases to the order of 3% of the total capillary flow when k_w is increased by ischemia.

CONCLUSION

An electronic network model for a tissue cylinder was postulated for the analysis of changes in COP appearing after transient occlusions of the LAD. The model was based on the Starling hypothesis and on volume elasticity of interstitial space. The characteristic time courses of COP changes suggest that the volume elasticity of local myocardium decreases and the fluid filtration coefficient of the capillary wall increases quickly during ischemia. Tissue fluid conductivity increases at the same time. These changes accelerate water accumulation in myocardial tissues and probably increase extravascular circulation, which may facilitate movements of macromolecules and the washout of metabolic wastes.

Present speculation includes many assumptions. Interstitial fluid oncotic pressure, tissue hydraulic pressure of myocardium, precise perfusion pressure and venous end pressure of the myocardial capillaries, and fluid conductivity through the gel of hyaluronic acid containing different amounts of water must be measured to obtain the decisive conclusions. Ingenious methods must be introduced in this area for the measurements of these important factors.

APPENDIX

Assuming that R_c, R_w, R_t, and C are constant in all sections, we obtain the following relations at point p in the model circuit (as illustrated in Fig. 4) by simple applications of Ohm's and Kirchhoff's law:

$$P_{p-1} - P_p = R_c I_{c_{p-1}}, \qquad [A1]$$

$$P_p - P_{p+1} = R_c I_{c_p}, \qquad [A2]$$

$$I_{c_{p-1}} - I_{c_p} = I_{w_p}, \qquad [A3]$$

$$I_{w_p} = 1/R_w(P_p - \alpha_p), \qquad [A4]$$

$$I_{wp} + I_{t_{p-1}} = I_{t_p} + I_{a_p},$$ [A5]

$$I_{a_p} = C \, d\alpha_p/dt,$$ [A6]

$$\alpha_{p-1} - \alpha_p = R_t I_{t_{p-1}},$$ [A7]

$$\alpha_p - \alpha_{p+1} = R_t I_{t_p}.$$ [A8]

In addition, the resistances and capacitance are expressed by using their specific values denoted with an asterisk and the length Δx as $R_c^* \, \Delta x$, $R_w^*/\Delta x$, $R_t^* \, \Delta x$, and $C^* \, \Delta x$.

Substraction of Eq. A2 from Eq. A1 and substitution for $(I_{c_{p-1}} - I_{c_p})$ according to Eqs. A3 and A4 yields the following equation:

$$P_{p-1} - 2P_p + P_{p+1} = (\Delta x)^2 \, R_c^*/R_w^* \, (P_p - \alpha_p).$$ [A9]

Subtraction of Eq. A7 from Eq. A8 is expressed by the following equation when rearranged using the relations in Eqs. A3 to A6 and specific values for resistances and capacitance:

$$\alpha_{p-1} - 2\alpha_p + \alpha_{p+1} = (\Delta x)^2 \left[R_t^* \, C^* \frac{d\alpha_p}{dt} - \frac{R_t^*}{R_w^*} (P_p - \alpha_p) \right].$$ [A10]

For the infinitely small Δx, Eqs. A9 and A10 become

$$\frac{\partial^2 P}{\partial x^2} = \frac{R_c^*}{R_w^*} (P - \alpha)$$ [A11]

and

$$\frac{\partial \alpha}{\partial t} = \frac{1}{R_t^* C^*} \frac{\partial^2 \alpha}{\partial x^2} + \frac{1}{R_w^* C^*} (P - \alpha).$$ [A12]

For the sake of simplicity, asterisks denoting specific values are omitted in the following description.

Pressures at the arterial end $(x = 0)$ and venous end $(x = L)$ of the capillary are P_{art} and P_v. If it is assumed that the water in the tissue cylinder does not move at the arterial and venous ends, no gradients in α exist there. These boundary conditions are written as follows:

for $x = 0$: $P = P_{art}$, $d\alpha/dx = 0$, [A13]

for $x = L$: $P = P_v$, $d\alpha/dx = 0$. [A14]

Integration of Eq. A12 in x yields the following equation:

$$\frac{\partial}{\partial t} \int_0^L \alpha \, dx = \frac{1}{R_t \cdot C} \int_0^L \frac{\partial^2 \alpha}{\partial x^2} \, dx + \frac{1}{R_w \cdot C} \int_0^L (P - \alpha) \, dx$$

$$= \frac{1}{R_t \cdot C} \frac{\partial \alpha}{\partial x} \Big|_0^L + \frac{L}{R_w \cdot C} (P_{av} - \alpha_{av}),$$ [A15]

where the subscript av indicates mean values of the variables along the x axis. Owing to Eqs. A13 and A14, Eq. A15 can simply be written as

$$\frac{\partial \alpha_{av}}{\partial t} = \frac{1}{R_w \cdot C} \cdot (P_{av} - \alpha_{av}).$$ [A16]

By assuming Eq. 3 and substituting $\alpha_{av} = e^{-t/R_w \cdot C} \cdot \alpha'$ into Eq. A16, we obtain Eq. 4.

REFERENCES

1. Fulton, W. F. M. (1964): The dynamic factor in enlargement of coronary arterial anastomoses. *Br. Heart J.,* 26:39–50.
2. Grabowski, E. F., and Bassingthwaighte, J. B. (1977): An osmotic weight transient model for estimation of capillary transport parameters in myocardium. In: *Microcirculation. Transport Mechanisms and Disease State 2,* edited by J. Grayson and W. Zingg, pp. 29–50. Plenum Press, New York.
3. Guyton, A. C. (1965): Interstitial fluid pressure. II. Pressure–volume curves of interstitial space. *Circ. Res.,* 16:452–460.
4. Guyton, A. C., Scheel, K., and Murphree, D. (1966): Interstitial fluid pressure. III. Its effects on resistance to tissue fluid mobility. *Circ. Res.,* 19:412–419.
5. Hansen, A. T. (1961): Osmotic pressure effect of the red blood cells—Possible physiological significance. *Nature,* 190:504–508.
6. Intaglietta, M. (1977): Transcapillary exchange of fluid in single microvessels. In: *Microcirculation. Volume 1,* edited by G. Kaley and B. M. Altura, pp. 197–212. University Park Press, Baltimore.
7. Intaglietta, M., and Zweifach, B. W. (1966): Indirect method for the measurement of pressure in blood capillaries. *Circ. Res.,* 19:199–208.
8. Koyama, T., Kakiuchi, Y., Sasajima, T., Makinoda, S., Arai, T., Ishikawa, M., and Nagashima, Ch. (1977): Water movement between myocardial tissue and capillary blood during and after coronary reactive hyperemia as studied by continuous measurement of colloid osmotic pressure of cardiac venous blood. *Experientia,* 33:1169–1170.
9. Koyama, T., Kikuchi, Y., and Kakiuchi, Y. (1979): An analysis of water movement between myocardial tissue and capillary blood during reactive hyperemia. *Jpn. J. Physiol.,* 29:1–13.
10. Landis, E. M., and Papenheimer, J. R. (1963): Exchanges of substances through the capillary walls. In: *Handbook of Physiology. Section II. Circulation 2,* edited by W. F. Hamilton and P. Dow, pp. 961–1034. American Physiological Society, Washington, D.C.
11. Oka, S., and Murata, T. (1970): A theoretical study of the flow of blood in capillary with permeable wall. *Jpn. J. Appl. Phys.,* 9:345–352.
12. Powell, W. J., Jr., DiBona, D. D., Fores, J., and Leaf, A. (1976): The protective effect of hyperosmotic mannitol in myocardial ischemia and necrosis. *Circulation,* 54:603–615.
13. Prather, J. W., Gaar, K. A., Jr., and Guyton, A. C. (1968): Direct continuous recording of plasma colloid osmotic pressure of whole blood. *J. Appl. Physiol.,* 24:602–605.
14. Smaje, L., Zweifach, B. W., and Intaglietta, M. (1970): Micropressure and capillary filtration coefficients in single vessels of the cremaster muscle of the rat. *Microvasc. Res.,* 3:96–110.
15. Starling, E. H. (1896): On the absorption of fluids from the connective tissue spaces. *J. Physiol. (Lond.),* 19:312–326.
16. Thews, G. (1962): Die sauerstoffdrucke im herzgewebe. *Pfuegers Arch.,* 276:166–181.
17. Vargas, F., and Johnson, J. A. (1967): Permeability of rabbit heart capillaries to nonelectrolytes. *Am. J. Physiol.,* 213:87–93.
18. Wiederhielm, C. A., Woodbury, J. W., Kirk, S., and Rushmer, R. F. (1964): Pulsatile pressure in the microcirculation of the frog's mesentery. *Am. J. Physiol.,* 207:173–176.
19. Winter, A. D., and Kruger, S. (1968): Drug effects on bulk flow through mesenteric membranes. *Arch. Int. Pharmacodyn. Ther.,* 173:213–225.

Ischemic Myocardium and Antianginal Drugs,
edited by M. M. Winbury and Y. Abiko.
Raven Press, New York © 1979.

Discussion: Structural and Biophysical Changes

Koroku Hashimoto, *Chairman*

Hashimoto: Before starting the discussion, I would like to make the definition of reversible changes clear. Dr. J. Schaper, will you please comment on this?

J. Schaper: My definition of reversible is based on ischemia ultrastructural changes, occurring mainly in mitochondria and nuclei. We obtained these criteria from animal experiments in which we compared resuscitability of the heart and functional and metabolic disturbances and the ability to recover with morphological changes.

Hashimoto: Thank you. Shall we open the discussion?

Winbury: I have two questions for Dr. Koyama. First, is there an effect of myocardial wall tension on the transport of water from the capillaries to the tissues? And second, what is the influence of changing the venous pressure on this transport? I am thinking in terms of the capillary filtration coefficient as measured by Folkow.

Koyama: I think that the extravascular compression on the capillary network plays a very important role in keeping the filtration coefficient at a constant level and that a decrease of the extravascular compression will initiate the flow of water from capillaries to the tissues. Unfortunately, we have no method by which we can measure the flow from capillaries to the tissue. For the second question, if the venous pressure is increased, the water filtration to the tissues will increase. According to the Starling hypothesis, an increase in the capillary pressure will increase the water filtration from the capillaries to the tissues.

Hashimoto: Dr. Jutta Schaper, do you have any comment on this? You have morphological findings observed 45 min after occlusion; the red cells had gone out of the vessels into the tissues.

J. Schaper: That's right.

Hashimoto: If you occlude the coronary artery for a very short period of time, do you find any expansion of interstitial space?

J. Schaper: Yes, we do. But I think it is very difficult to compare the results between the experiment with longer occlusion to that with shorter occlusion because the effects of coronary ligation on the myocardium also depend on the oxygen consumption of the heart. In those experiments, where no pretreatment with propranolol or anything else had been done, we saw, after various periods of time, the passage of fluid into the extravascular space.

Hashimoto: Do you find swelling of the endothelial cells?

J. Schaper: Yes, that may occur.

W. Schaper: I would like to add to that comment. It really depends very much on the oxygen consumption of the heart during the occlusion. We have found that a few minutes of occlusion at a very high oxygen consumption will produce all these changes that have been presented. On the other hand, at a very depressed oxygen consumption of about 4 to 5 ml/min/100 g of tissue, you find nothing at all after 3 hr. The tissue is fully viable when the oxygen consumption is that low.

Hashimoto: Isn't time very important in this kind of experiment?

W. Schaper: I think that we have three determinants of reversible or irreversible injury. These are time, oxygen consumption, and collateral blood flow.

Bing: Dr. Jutta Schaper, I have two questions on your paper. First, were the inclusion bodies that you demonstrated more numerous after reperfusion? According to various people, calcium goes into the cells as a consequence of reperfusion. Is there an increase in those inclusion bodies? Second, I also would like to ask you about the fatty droplets. You have really found what is an equivalent of the metabolic changes that have been observed with the accumulation of free fatty acids in the heart muscle in ischemia. So, I just wanted to know, what relationship was there between reperfusion and these elements?

J. Schaper: After 15 min of reperfusion, many more cells contain these inclusion bodies, which most probably are an accumulation of calcium, phosphate, protein, and lipids, all put together. And these are much more numerous after reperfusion than after ischemia alone.

Bing: Do you think they are calcium phosphate or what?

J. Schaper: All of them are; certainly calcium and a large amount of phosphate, also some proteins and some lipids are present.

Bleifeld: Would you like to comment about the changes in relation to the region of myocardium, i.e., endo- and epicardial changes? And second, do you think either the amount of collateral blood flow or the pressure plays any role?

J. Schaper: There are big differences between the endocardial and the epicardial tissue samples. Most of the epicardial tissue samples show only a slight and reversible injury (i.e., the injury is completely reversed after 15 min of reperfusion), whereas the endocardium shows more pronounced damage after ischemia that becomes even more severe during reperfusion. I think my husband can answer the next question better than I can.

W. Schaper: Is this the question about the amount of collateral flow?

Bleifeld: Yes, the amount of flow and possibly the pressure by which this flow is delivered to the myocardium.

W. Schaper: You mean perfusion pressure?

Bleifeld: Yes.

W. Schaper: There is a linear relationship between collateral blood flow and aortic perfusion pressure. So the higher the perfusion pressure is, the more collateral flow and the less ischemic damage would be expected.

Bleifeld: I suppose collateral vascular beds are preformed in the acute state. Is that right?

W. Schaper: That is true.

Bleifeld: The amount of collateral blood flow in a given situation is dependent on the level of the aortic perfusion pressure.

Opie: I just want to continue with Dr. Bleifeld's line of questioning because a lot of us are oriented toward the metabolic aspects of reperfusion—the calcium phenomenon, oxygen toxicity, and that sort of thing. I wonder if we should also consider another relation between coronary flow and metabolism that Arnold and Lochner showed years ago in Germany and that we also showed independently in London. This is related to the questionable phenomenon of Gregg, that in some way the coronary flow or pressure may be determining the oxygen uptake of the heart, rather than the other way around. I feel this is relevant to your question, Dr. Bleifeld, about whether the degree of flow or the pressure of the flow could, in some way, be determining the metabolism.

Henry: I have a question for Dr. J. Schaper. I noticed an absence of I-bands and invaginations of nuclear membranes after 90 min of ischemia without reperfusion. Are these changes attributable to the fixation procedure used?

J. Schaper: Yes, they were immersion fixed. I called it normal pattern because this is the normal pattern of myocardial cells in immersion-fixed tissues. We have light I-bands in immersion-fixed tissues only after a very long period of ischemia and severe or irreversible damage.

Myocardial Blood Flow

Ischemic Myocardium and Antianginal Drugs,
edited by M. M. Winbury and Y. Abiko.
Raven Press, New York © 1979.

Stenosis: Regional Myocardial Ischemia and Reserve

Martin M. Winbury and *Burton B. Howe

Office of Scientific Affairs, Warner-Lambert Company, Morris Plains, New Jersey 07950

Stenosis of large coronary arteries affects not only the coronary blood flow rate of the left ventricle but also the transmural distribution of that flow when the stenosis becomes critical (1,7,13). Usually, the autoregulatory reserve of the left ventricle in normal dog and normal man is considerable. In the absence of a marked degree of coronary artery disease or stenosis, the coronary blood flow rate of the left ventricle can increase from three- to fivefold during stress such as that imposed by severe exercise or during reactive hyperemia following coronary occlusion for a period as short as 15 sec. The autoregulatory reserve will permit the maintenance of normal blood flow until there is a greater than 90% reduction in a cross-sectional area of the lumen of the vessel. At such a point there is maximal arteriolar dilatation, and the flow is now pressure dependent and sensitive to any slight change in stenosis resistance (16). A further decrease in luminal size will cause a marked decrease in basal blood flow.

In order to determine appropriately the coronary reserve, it is necessary to stress the myocardium and/or increase the rate of blood flow by producing maximal arteriolar vasodilatation (5,8). This can be accomplished by stress such as exercise or tachycardia, as is done in the evaluation of patients. Under those circumstances, blood flow is adequate at rest, and there is no evidence of coronary insufficiency. However, during stress, stenosis may become flow limiting, and coronary insufficiency with the clinical signs of angina pectoris can develop. Hyperemia can also be produced by coronary occlusion or by use of potent coronary arteriolar dilators such as adenosine, dipyridamole, and carbochromen. When the stenosis reaches the critical point, the stress flow response will be less than normal because vasodilator reserve has been exhausted as a result of the arteriolar vasodilatation distal to the stenosis. This usually occurs when there is a reduction in the lumen greater than 45% (3–5,8). Beyond this point, a further decrease in lumen size or a decrease in peripheral coronary pressure will cause a decrease in maximal coronary blood flow. Thus, it is necessary to produce maximal vasodilatation in order to evaluate and determine the stenosis reserve.

---

* Present address: ICI—United States, Inc., Wilmington, Delaware 19897.

It is well known that the subendocardial region (endo) of the left ventricle is more vulnerable than the subepicardial region (epi) to any form of stress, and from this it has been inferred that the vasodilator reserve of the subendocardial region is less than that of the subepicardium (9,14). Perfusion through the left ventricle wall appears to be homogeneous, with the endo and the epi equal or the endo somewhat higher (1,6,9,10). Approximately 85% of the coronary flow occurs during diastole because of the extravascular compression and wall tension developed during systole, particularly in the deeper region. The remaining 15% that occurs during systole is confined primarily to the epi, and all the blood flow to the endo takes place during the diastolic period (9). Accordingly, there is a gradient of vascular tone, with the endo having a greater conductance than the epi since all the flow in that region must take place during diastole. If we assume that the vascular beds of each of the regions are relatively similar in size, it is evident that the autoregulatory reserve of the endo is smaller than that of the epi.

Among the factors that influence the effect of stenosis are (a) the *reduction in luminal size* (reactive hyperemia disappears when there is an 80% decrease); (b) the *length of the stenosis* (2,8), which will not be considered in this report; (c) the *pressure gradient* at rest and during reactive hyperemia (at low flow rates, the pressure gradient does not appear to increase with flow unless the stenosis is extreme; however, at high flow rates, the pressure gradient increases rapidly with the increase in flow rate); (d) *peripheral coronary pressure* at rest and during reactive hyperemia (this is important in the distribution of blood flow since the diastolic perfusion gradient is critical for perfusion of the endo; with stenosis, high velocity flow decreases peripheral coronary pressure and favors perfusion of the epi); (e) *vasodilator reserve* in each region (it is lower in the endo); (f) *flow rate through the stenosis,* which affects the pressure gradient and the peripheral coronary pressure for perfusion (as the flow rate increases, the pressure gradient increases and peripheral coronary pressure decreases); (g) the *gradient of wall tension,* which is greatest in the endo; and (h) the *gradient of arteriolar tone,* which is lower in the endo and is related to the vasodilator reserve.

The purpose of these studies was to quantitate the vasodilator reserve in the endo and epi and to determine changes in the pressure gradient and perfusion that occur with varying degrees of stenosis. The first phase of these studies involved determination of changes in tissue oxygen tension in the endo and epi, as well as in reactive hyperemia at varying degrees of stenosis. The second phase was to determine the changes in regional perfusion based on hydrogen clearance. Finally, the third phase was the determination of peripheral pressures and pressure gradients and resistances at various degrees of stenosis.

In general, our studies showed that in the normal dog endo, autoregulatory reserve is exhausted at a peripheral diastolic perfusion pressure distal to the stenosis of about 70 mm Hg. On the other hand, the epi reserve is maintained until diastolic perfusion pressure decreases to about 40 mm Hg. Another finding of interest from these studies is the fact that the pressure curve crosses the zero intercept for flow at a positive value of somewhere in the range of 20 mm Hg, and it is suggested that critical closing in the subendocardium occurs at an average of about 30 mm Hg and then in the subepicardium at about 12 to 18 mm Hg.

In spite of the fact that transmural perfusion is homogeneous, there is a gradient of oxygen tension, with the endo one-half to two-thirds of epi, and of carbon dioxide, with the endo higher (14,15). Furthermore, metabolic studies demonstrate that the endo tends to become anaerobic more readily than the epi when blood flow or perfusion pressure is diminished. Accordingly, this suggests that the balance between supply and demand for oxygen and substrates is more critical in the endo because of the low reserve in supply and that, with stress, the endo will become hypoxic and tend toward anaerobic metabolism.

METHODS

We used mongrel dogs of either sex weighing between 18 and 30 kg. Animals were anesthetized with pentobarbital sodium (30 mg/kg i.v.); supplemental anesthesia was used as required. The left carotid artery was ligated and the central end cannulated with a large bore polyethylene catheter (PE 320) filled with a 1% heparin saline solution. The catheter was advanced into the aortic arch and connected to a Statham high pressure transducer (P 23DB). A cuffed endotracheal tube was inserted into the trachea for subsequent artificial respiration. The right femoral vein was catheterized with a small bore polyethylene catheter (PE 190) for administration of drugs and supplemental anesthetic.

At this stage, the animals were artificially respired with a Harvard dual-phase respiration pump. The respiration rate usually was between 14 and 18 strokes/min. The volume of each cycle was adjusted after the chest was opened to adequately inflate the lung and yet not interfere with venous return and/or cause changes in the heart position. The left side of the chest was opened in the fifth intercostal space and a pericardial cradle prepared to expose the anterior surface from base to apex. A 1- to 1.5-cm region of the left anterior descending artery was isolated by blunt dissection approximately one-fourth to one-half of the distance between the base and the apex for placement of a flow probe, a hydraulic occluder, and a snare from the central to the distal end. The inner diameter of the flow probe was between 1.5 and 2 mm and was chosen to fit snugly around the blood vessel without producing any degree of stenosis but providing continuous contact between the blood vessel wall and the inner surface of the flow probe. Mean coronary blood flow, as well as phasic flow, was measured with a Biotronex (BL-610) pulsed logic flowmeter. The hydraulic occluder (Rhodes Medical Instruments, Inc., 21044 Ventura Boulevard, Woodland Hills, Ca. 91364), which was 3 mm in length, was placed around the vessel distal to the flow probe and in such a position that the occluder, when inflated, did not interfere with the function of the flow probe. The occluder consisted of a latex balloon inside a rigid plastic outer container. Gradual occlusion of the vessel was accomplished by filling the latex balloon with liquid. The balloon and the attached tubing were initially filled with saline. The tubing was connected to a 1-ml tuberculin syringe by a needle cemented to the syringe, which was also filled with fluid. Movement of the syringe was via a micrometer screw holder which enabled gradual and reproducible degrees of inflation of the balloon and, thereby, reproducible reductions in blood flow by gradual stenosis. Zero flow was produced by total occlusion with a snare occluder. This snare was distal to the balloon occluder and consisted of either fine umbilical tape or a ligature that was passed underneath the vessel and through a length of polyethylene tubing. Total occlusion was produced by pulling on the ligature or the umbilical tape.

Following these general procedures, animals were used for studies on regional oxygen tension (14), regional perfusion by H_2 clearance (6,10), or peripheral coronary pressure in the vessel distal to the flow probe. Peripheral coronary pressure was measured in the following manner. Pressure in the left anterior descending coronary artery (LAD) distal to a stenosis was measured with a short 20-gauge teflon catheter filled with 1% heparin saline solution. A small branch of approximately 0.5 mm of the LAD near the apex of the heart was isolated, and two ligatures were placed beneath the vessel. The distal ligature was tied and a small incision was made central to the tie. The catheter was inserted into the central end and the proximal ligature was tied carefully around the catheter. Care was taken to avoid occlusion of the catheter. If the branch was not along the main stream of the LAD, the catheter was gently manipulated to the LAD and used for measurement of peripheral coronary pressure after connecting the distal end to the high pressure transducer (P 23DB). The aortic transducer and the peripheral coronary pressure transducer were calibrated simultaneously with a single hydraulic system, and pressures were measured simultaneously throughout the experiment. Thus the pressure gradient across the stenosis was obtained continuously, as well as aortic pressure and peripheral coronary pressure. These values were measured in five animals; in an additional three animals, regional oxygen tension in the subendocardium and subepicardium was studied simultaneously with the changes in pressures.

RESULTS

There were three phases to these investigations as described in the methods. Because the results on tissue oxygen tension and perfusion are quite similar, they will be described together in the first section. The results on peripheral perfusion pressure, pressure gradients, and resistances will be considered separately, although we may make reference to these findings in the first section.

The studies confirm those of many others that the subendocardium is more vulnerable to ischemia and hypoxia than the subepicardium when the perfusion pressure and blood supply are compromised. There is an inappropriate distribution of blood flow owing to the more rapid decline of the endo perfusion gradient (9,10,14,15). Graded stenosis of a coronary artery leads to a more rapid decline in basal oxygen tension and perfusion in the endo than in the epi (15). Stenosis has a more profound effect on blood flow and the distribution of flow during maximal vasodilatation. Thus the transmural differences in perfusion and oxygen tension are accentuated during maximal arteriolar dilatation following release of a coronary occlusion (reactive hyperemia) or after administration of chromonar (carbochromen). Vasodilator reserve or autoregulation is exhausted by a smaller reduction of perfusion pressure and flow in the endo than in the epi. Finally, during maximal vasodilatation, the resistance across the stenosis is a critical determinant of blood flow and its transmural distribution.

Oxygen Tension and Perfusion

Changes in Basal Values with Changes in Blood Flow

The transmural gradient in oxygen tension (Po_2) is obvious from Fig. 1. Basal epi Po_2 of 27.1 Torr was approximately 1.3 times endo Po_2 of 21 Torr.

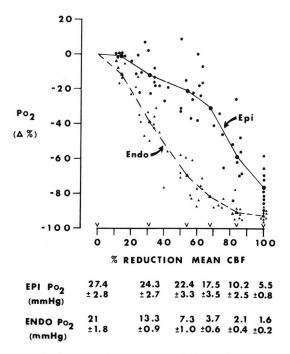

EPI Po_2 (mmHg)	27.4 ± 2.8	24.3 ± 2.7	22.4 ± 3.3	17.5 ± 3.5	10.2 ± 2.5	5.5 ± 0.8
ENDO Po_2 (mmHg)	21 ± 1.8	13.3 ± 0.9	7.3 ± 1.0	3.7 ± 0.6	2.1 ± 0.4	1.6 ± 0.2

FIG. 1. Relationship of changes in subepicardial *(epi)* and subendocardial *(endo)* oxygen tension (Po_2) to changes in mean coronary blood flow (CBF). CBF reduced by stepwise stenosis as indicated by symbols on CBF scale. Mean values for Po_2 are given in table at bottom for control and five steps of diminished flow. Note the linear decline in endo Po_2 and the two-phase decline in epi Po_2 with reduction in mean CBF. *Circles,* epi; *triangles,* endo.

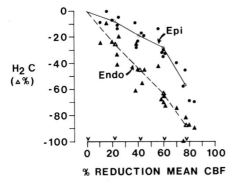

CBF (ml/min/100g)	80 ±5.5	62 ±3.4	47 ±3.2	33 ±2	18 ±1.1
C EPI (ml/min/100g)	97 ±8.6	90 ±6.1	79 ±6.9	70 ±5.9	41 ±5.6
C ENDO (ml/min/100g)	87 ±4.2	67 ±5.2	48 ±7.3	32 ±5.6	12 ±4

FIG. 2. Relationship of changes in epi *(circles)* and endo *(triangles)* perfusion (H_2 C—hydrogen clearance) to changes in mean CBF. Mean values for CBF and epi and endo perfusion are given in table at bottom for increasing degrees of stenosis. Note linear decline in endo perfusion and two-stage decline in epi perfusion.

On the other hand, transmural perfusion was homogeneous with an epi/endo ratio of 1.1. Basal coronary blood flow (CBF) and epi and endo perfusion values were 80, 97, and 87 ml/min/100 g, respectively (Fig. 2).

Although there were several degrees of stenosis prior to the 0 point on the blood flow scale (mean CBF) in Figs. 1 and 2, there were no reductions in Po_2 or perfusion because the stenosis was less than "critical."

Oxygen Tension

Graded reductions in CBF were accompanied by a steep linear decline in endo Po_2, as illustrated in Fig. 1. When CBF was reduced 60%, Po_2 was down about 80% from a resting value of 21 Torr to about 5 to 6 Torr. Following this, the decline was more gradual. At zero flow, endo Po_2 was between 1 and 2 Torr.

Basal epi Po_2 declined in two major phases. The first was gradual, and a 70% decline in CBF produced only a 30% decline in Po_2. But beyond that point, epi Po_2 declined sharply with a slope comparable to that of endo Po_2.

Perfusion

Figure 2 shows that the relative change in endo perfusion with CBF was linear with a slope close to 1. At 85% decrease in CBF endo perfusion was zero, suggesting a critical closing. Epi perfusion declined in two stages as did Po_2. Between 0 and 60% decrease in CBF, epi perfusion declined 30%. The second phase was similar to that of the endo. Epi perfusion ceased when flow was reduced 100%. The table at the bottom of Fig. 2 shows the close correspondence between the absolute values of the average CBF (flowmeter) and endo perfusion (ENDO), which suggests that the electrode placed at a depth of 9 mm in the left ventricular free wall samples a region that represents a large mass of the wall. The epi/endo perfusion ratio increased from a control of 1.11 to 4.45 when blood flow was diminished by 78%.

The parallelism between changes in regional perfusion (Fig. 2) and changes in regional Po_2 (Fig. 1) with changes in CBF is obvious, even to the break in the epi curve at a CBF reduction of greater than 60%. It can be assumed that during the first phase, epi autoregulation was still capable of compensating, to some extent, for the decline in CBF (and perfusion pressure), and thus it attenuated the decline in Po_2 and perfusion. At a reduction in CBF of more than 60%, epi reserve was exhausted; endo reserve was exhausted at a 0 to 10% reduction in CBF.

Effect of Stepwise Stenosis on Regional Oxygen Tension and Perfusion—Estimation of Epi and Endo Reserve

CBF at rest or under basal conditions will not indicate an impairment of perfusion or diminution of reserve until the lumen area of the artery supplying the region is reduced beyond a critical point of 90% (4,12). However, during maximal vasodilatation, the critical reduction in the lumen area is about 70%. Beyond that point, CBF during maximal vasodilatation will be pressure dependent and will decrease with a further reduction in vessel lumen, but basal CBF will not be affected. Therefore, it was necessary to determine the effect of graded degrees of stenosis on maximal CBF during reactive hyperemia (RH), as well as on basal CBF and basal regional Po_2 or perfusion. The RH response will indicate changes in overall autoregulatory reserve, and basal regional Po_2 or perfusion will indicate regional reserve.

An example of the effect of progressive stenosis on Po_2 is illustrated in Fig. 3. Prior to panel A of Fig. 3, the vessel was gradually occluded but to less than the "critical" point. Panel A represents the normal value. A 15-sec total occlusion produced a slight transient decline in endo Po_2 and no change in epi Po_2 and maximal RH (overshoot of CBF). Responses were similar at smaller degrees of stenosis (not shown). An increase in stenosis to reduce RH by 50% (panel B) did not alter basal CBF or Po_2 or the fall in endo Po_2, but it prolonged recovery time. Stenosis that reduced RH 85 to 90% (panel C) further increased recovery time of endo Po_2 but did not alter basal levels of Po_2 or CBF. Epi Po_2 now showed a rise and fall during occlusion and a marked overshoot following release of the occlusion. Basal endo Po_2 declined when CBF was reduced by 20% (panel D), but basal epi Po_2 was still maintained and a slight RH response was still present; endo reserve was exhausted. Further stenosis to reduce basal CBF 50% (panel E) caused a decline in epi Po_2, further decreased endo Po_2, and abolished RH; epi reserve was now exhausted.

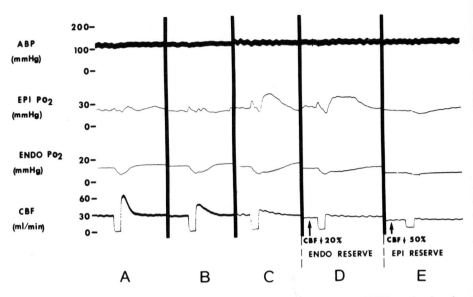

FIG. 3. Effect of increasing stenosis on CBF, RH, aortic blood pressure (ABP), and epi and endo Po_2. The first stage *(panel A)* serves as control since the stenosis had no effect. Subsequent stages reduced RH. Endo reserve was exhausted (basal Po_2 decreased) in the fourth stage *(panel D)*, and epi reserve was exhausted in the fifth *(panel E)*.

Pattern of Changes in Autoregulatory Reserve in Endo and Epi Po_2

The overall pattern based on Po_2 changes is shown in Fig. 4. The RH response (shaded area between resting CBF and RH flow) is an index of overall autoregulatory reserve, and the basal epi and endo Po_2 show when regional reserve was exhausted. Stenosis of the LAD was increased until RH started to decline. This came more from endo reserve than epi reserve since endo but not epi Po_2 declined during the 15-sec occlusion, as shown in Fig. 3. When CBF was reduced about 10% and RH about 80%, endo reserve was exhausted because the next stage of stenosis caused endo Po_2 to decline. Epi reserve was exhausted when stenosis reduced resting CBF 50% and almost abolished RH. This corresponds to about 95% stenosis.

Perfusion

These experiments were similar to those on Po_2 described above, except regional reserve was based on H_2 clearance (Fig. 5). RH following a 15-sec occlusion was determined after graded steps of stenosis. In addition, basal endo and epi perfusion were measured. The overall results illustrated in Fig. 5 agree closely with those for endo and epi reserve based on Po_2 in Fig. 4. The gradual steps of stenosis that produced no effect on the variables are not illustrated in the figure; we start with the critical point beyond which RH was diminished.

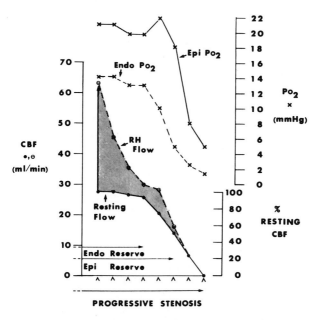

FIG. 4. Effect of progressive stenosis on CBF at rest and during reactive hyperemia (RH) and epi and endo Po_2. Overall coronary reserve is indicated by *shaded area* between resting and RH flow. Each increasing stage of stenosis is indicated by symbol on lowest scale. Endo reserve was exhausted at the fourth stage and epi was exhausted at the sixth stage.

RH was more sensitive to stenosis than were resting regional perfusion or resting CBF. As in the previous figure, RH is represented by the shaded area. Basal endo and epi perfusion and CBF were equal and unchanged (87 to 94 ml/min/100 g) through the four degrees of increasing stenosis, even though RH decreased from 378 to 30 ml/min/100 g or about 92% of the peak control RH (peak control RH = RH CBF − resting CBF). This was the limit of endo reserve since subsequent stenosis decreased endo perfusion and resting CBF. Epi reserve was exhausted at the seventh stage of stenosis shown in Fig. 5. At that point, epi perfusion was reduced slightly, RH abolished, and endo perfusion and CBF reduced 45%. Beyond this point, further stenosis caused a parallel decrease in epi and endo perfusion and in CBF. In agreement with Fig. 2, epi perfusion persisted at a low value when endo perfusion was zero.

The critical points for exhaustion of endo reserve and epi reserve based on regional perfusion are almost equal to those based on regional Po_2. Endo reserve was exhausted when RH was reduced by 80 to 90% and CBF was almost unchanged, and epi reserve was exhausted when RH was abolished and CBF was down 45 to 50%.

On the basis of Figs. 3 to 5, it can be concluded that the autoregulatory reserve of the endo is far smaller than that of the epi. Nonetheless, under resting conditions in the open chest dog, the reserve is extensive and stenosis first

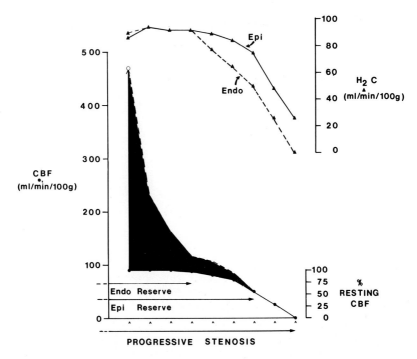

FIG. 5. Effect of progressive stenosis on CBF at rest and during RH and epi and endo perfusion (H_2 C—hydrogen clearance). Overall coronary reserve is indicated by *shaded area*. Endo and epi reserves are indicated by *horizontal lines with arrow*.

affects high-flow states (RH) and then low-flow states (resting CBF). Stenosis resistance becomes flow limiting when reserve is exhausted (11,16).

Effect of Acute Occlusion

Oxygen Tension

In Fig. 3 we showed that in the absence of stenosis, a 10- to 15-sec occlusion had little effect on epi Po_2. Therefore, total occlusion was maintained for 1 to 3 min (Fig. 6). The duration of occlusion does not appear to be a factor in the peak RH flow, but it does influence the duration of RH. However, regional Po_2 is more sensitive to the duration. Epi Po_2 does not decline to a minimal value unless the occlusion is maintained for at least 1 min. The onset of the fall in endo Po_2 is immediate, but it is delayed for as long as 20 sec for epi Po_2. Furthermore, the rate of fall is sharper in endo Po_2. Finally, endo Po_2 declines more than 90%, but epi Po_2 is more variable and may range from no change to 80%.

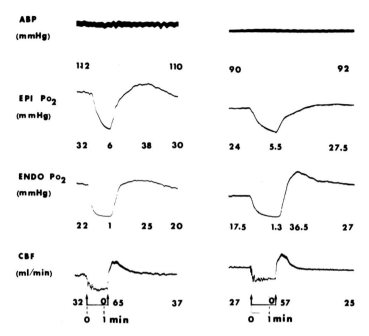

FIG. 6. Effect of acute occlusion and subsequent RH on epi and endo Po_2. Numbers represent values for ABP, Po_2, or CBF. Example on *left* shows no overshoot of Po_2; that on the *right* demonstrates overshoot of endo Po_2 during RH.

Following release of the occlusion, there is always an overshoot of CBF (RH), but regional Po_2 may or may not show an overshoot (see Fig. 6). Endo Po_2 starts to rise before and more rapidly than epi Po_2.

Perfusion

The animal was switched from breathing 2% H_2 to breathing room air during the period prior to occlusion in some of the studies and during the occlusion period in others. In the former case (Fig. 7), it was possible to determine endo and epi perfusion during the control period, total occlusion, and the peak steady state RH from the same clearance curve. The duration of occlusion was from 1.5 to 2.5 min to produce a long period of steady state maximal RH flow to permit a monoexponential clearance curve of sufficient duration for calculation of the perfusion rate.

An example of an acute occlusion followed by release and RH is shown in Fig. 7. The clearance started prior to occlusion shows the decline in the H_2 current, which ceased during occlusion. In some animals, epi perfusion continued at a low level during occlusion, but endo perfusion invariably dropped to zero. The increased perfusion during reactive hyperemia is apparent from the increased

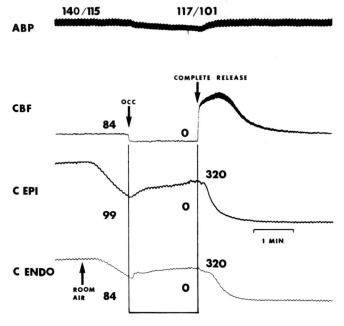

FIG. 7. Effect of acute occlusion and subsequent RH on epi and endo perfusion. Numbers represent values for ABP, CBF, and perfusion (C). Values for blood flow and perfusion are in milligrams per minute per 100 g. Peak CBF during RH is 400 ml/min/100 g. The record for epi and endo C represents H_2 desaturation curves from intramyocardial polarographic recordings.

slope of the H_2 washout. This is in contrast to the Po_2 changes, which are variable and do not show a consistent overshoot. The increased CBF and regional perfusion is a result of arteriolar autoregulation.

The difference between the response of Po_2 and perfusion during RH is obvious from comparison of Figs. 6 and 7. This is neither an artifact nor is it anatomical (e.g., interarterial anastomoses). Rather it is probably physiological, since tissue Po_2 is determined not only by the supply of oxygen (perfusion), but also by the regional oxygen requirement. During the occlusion period an oxygen debt is accumulated, and it is repaid by the autoregulatory increase in blood flow. However, the additional oxygen supply is utilized for the resynthesis of intermediates utilized during the anaerobic period. Consequently, tissue Po_2 may not parallel tissue perfusion.

Partial Release After Acute or Gradual Occlusion

The objective of these studies was to determine the effect of restricting RH flow to the CBF level encountered during the control period prior to occlusion. This provides information on the effect of stenosis on the transmural distribution

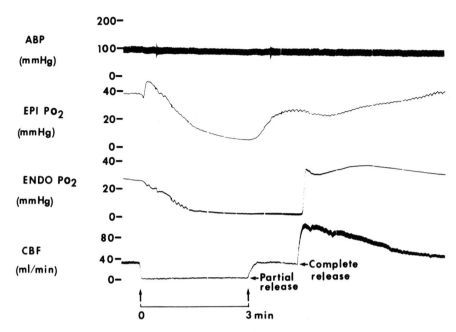

FIG. 8. Effect of restricted reflow following total occlusion on epi and endo Po_2. During partial release, stenosis maintained CBF at a preocclusion level. There was no stenosis at complete release. Note the lack of change in endo Po_2, but the rise in epi Po_2 on partial release.

of blood flow during maximal vasodilatation of the arterioles in the epi and the endo.

Oxygen Tension

Figure 8 shows the effect of partially releasing the occlusion just enough to permit CBF to return to the preocclusion control level and to prevent RH (partial release). Endo Po_2 did not change from the minimal occlusion value, but epi Po_2 returned to almost 70% of the control. This is an example of "coronary steal" or inappropriate distribution of blood flow. When the stenosis was removed (complete release), RH occurred, endo Po_2 rose sharply to greater than control values, and epi Po_2 rose more gradually.

A similar pattern was observed when the occlusion was produced by stepwise stenosis. Partial release permitted a slight rise in endo Po_2 (1.4 to 5 Torr) but a significant rise in epi Po_2 (5 to 17 Torr). Complete release of the stenosis was followed by RH and overshoot of epi and endo Po_2.

Perfusion

In this study (Fig. 9), the animal was switched from H_2 to room air during the acute occlusion phase (room air); no perfusion was observed. When the

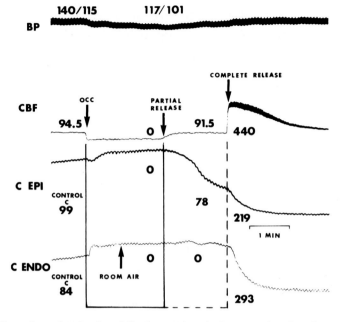

FIG. 9. Effect of restricted reflow following total occlusion on epi and endo perfusion (C). Values for CBF and perfusion are in milliliters per minute per 100 g. During partial release, stenosis maintained CBF at a preocclusion level. Note the lack of change in endo C, but the rise in epi C on partial release. Both were increased during the hyperemia following complete release of the stenosis.

occlusion was reduced to restore blood flow to the control value, epi perfusion increased to about 80% of the control value, but endo perfusion remained at zero. Studies from a large number of animals show that epi perfusion always increased during partial release but not above the control rate; however, endo perfusion did not increase. When the stenosis was removed, the normal RH occurred.

These studies demonstrate that restriction of blood flow by stenosis during maximal vasodilatation produced inappropriate distribution of blood flow across the left ventricular wall with underperfusion of the subendocardium. In the subsequent section, we will show that this occurred as a result of reduced peripheral coronary pressure that was inadequate for perfusion of the deeper regions.

Peripheral Coronary Pressure and Stenosis Gradient

Perfusion pressure distal to the stenosis is determined by the pressure central to the stenosis, the degree of stenosis, the blood flow rate, and the resistance of the arteriolar bed distal to the stenosis (3,4,12,16). The pressure gradient across the stenosis also varies with these same factors and stenosis resistance is not a constant for a fixed reduction in lumen size but increases with the velocity of flow. These points will be demonstrated by the experiments described in the subsequent sections.

Relationship of Blood Flow to Peripheral Coronary Pressure and Pressure Gradient

Figure 10A describes the relationship of CBF at rest and during peak RH to peripheral coronary pressure (PCP) and pressure gradient (PG). The changes in these variables were produced by progressive stenosis of the LAD. PCP is the horizontal scale, and PG is the value at each point on the resting CBF and RH line.

Certain major points can be observed in the lower portion of Fig. 10A. RH flow (dashed line) was considerably more sensitive than resting CBF to decreases in perfusion pressure. At a fixed degree of stenosis, PCP was lower and PG was greater during the increased flow of RH than at resting CBF (each set of points on the resting and RH graphs connected by a thin line represents a different fixed degree of stenosis). CBF crossed the PCP line at pressure between 13 and 20 Torr; this corresponds to critical closing.

In the upper portion of Fig. 10A, it can be observed that calculated small vessel resistance (RS) at rest decreased until RH disappeared (autoregulation), whereas RS during RH increased as PCP diminished.

Resting CBF did not change markedly until resting PCP had been reduced below 60 mm Hg and resting PG exceeded 40 mm Hg. RH flow declined more rapidly with the increase in stenosis; this was accompanied by a greater PG and lower PCP than at resting CBF. RH disappeared (autoregulatory reserve was exhausted) when PCP was 40 to 50 mm Hg and the corresponding gradient 70 to 60 mm Hg. Beyond this point, stenosis resistance was limiting to flow. Coronary flow was reduced to zero at a critical closing pressure ranging between 13 to 20 mm Hg.

Distal coronary RS is due to the resistance of the arteriolar bed distal to the stenosis. This decreased to less than 70% of control until PCP declined below 40 mm Hg, at which point there was an increase. RS during RH increased gradually until a PCP of 50 mm Hg; then the rise was rapid. This is probably due to left ventricular wall tension on the endo and the epi with critical closing. It has been estimated that the percentage decrease in lumen corresponds to the following PCP values: 80 Torr, 84%; 50 Torr, 92%; 40 Torr, 93%; and 22 Torr, 95% (4,15).

Chromonar produces maximal coronary arteriolar dilatation equivalent to peak RH and has a long duration of effect. Thus flow is pressure dependent, and the change in total resistance is due to the stenosis resistance. The pressure–flow relationship in Fig. 10B is identical to that during RH in Fig. 10A. These were obtained in the same animal. Critical closing was quite similar. The change in RS with the decrease in PCP in Fig. 10B also parallels the RS–PCP curve during RH in Fig. 10A.

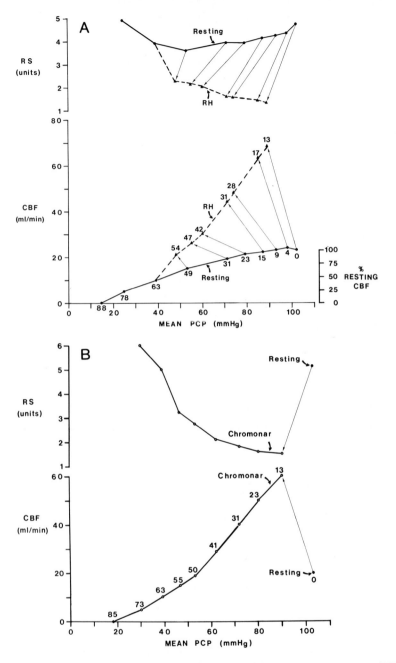

FIG. 10. Relationship of coronary blood flow (CBF) to peripheral coronary pressure (PCP) at rest and during maximal vasodilatation. **A:** CBF at rest *(solid line)* and during RH *(dashed line)*. The pressure gradient (PG) across the stenosis is given at each point on the CBF lines. The thin lines with the arrows connecting points from the resting to RH CBF curves shows the changes in PCP and PG at a given degree of stenosis. PG is greater and PCP lower at the higher flow rates of RH. Zero flow crosses the pressure axis at 18 mm Hg. Distal bed resistance (RS) at rest and during RH is shown in the upper section of the figure. **B:** CBF during maximal vasodilatation due to chromonar. This curve is very similar to the RH curve in Fig. 10A.

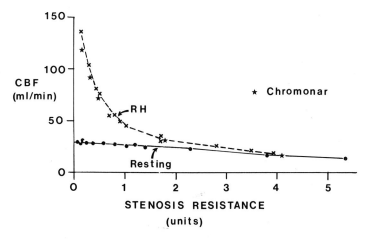

FIG. 11. Relationship of CBF to stenosis resistance at rest *(circles)* and during RH *(crosses)* or chromonar vasodilatation *(stars)*. Note marked effect of stenosis resistance on high CBF rates.

Relationship of Stenosis Resistance to Flow at Rest and During RH or Chromonar

Figure 11 describes the relationship of resting stenosis resistance (SR) to CBF at rest and during maximal flow due to RH or chromonar. In our calculations there was only one SR value for each degree of stenosis, since resting PG and resting CBF values were used (resting PG/resting CBF). Figure 11 shows that higher flow rates (during RH and chromonar) are more influenced by a decrease in lumen than are low flow rates (resting), which is in agreement with others (11,16). Thus RH and chromonar CBF declined rapidly with increasing SR, but there was only a small effect on resting CBF.

Actually, SR is dependent not only on the radius of the vessel lumen but also on the flow velocity. Therefore, SR calculated as PG/CBF for a particular lumen size increases with flow at high flow rates, such as those during RH or chromonar; at low flow rates, however, SR is relatively constant. This suggests laminar flow at low flow rates, and turbulence, flow separation, or entrance effects at high flow rates (12).

Overall Relationship of PG to Po_2, Regional Reserve, Resistance, and Perfusion Pressure

The effect of increasing degrees of stenosis on endo and epi Po_2, CBF, and pressures was determined simultaneously in several animals. The results of these studies are depicted in Fig. 12. The pattern of change in Po_2, basal CBF, and RH CBF is similar to that of Fig. 3. Endo reserve was exhausted at the third degree of stenosis. At that time mean PCP, diastolic pressure, and PG were 90, 70, and 19 Torr, respectively; CBF was reduced 11% and RH 82%. Epi

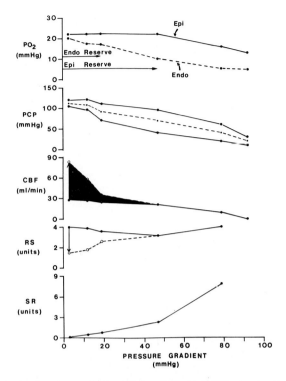

FIG. 12. Relationship of pressure gradient to Po_2, PCP, and CBF at rest and during hyperemia, RS at rest *(solid line)* and during RH *(dashed line)* and stenosis resistance (SR). Endo reserve was exhausted at diastolic PCP of 70 mm Hg and epi reserve at 40 mm Hg.

reserve was exhausted at the fourth degree of stenosis. Corresponding values were 70, 40, and 47 Torr and 25% and 100%, respectively. Small vessel RS at rest decreased to a minimum of 64% when RH was abolished. RS during RH increased, as did SR. The pressure gradients at various percentages of stenosis were 20 Torr at 84% stenosis; 40 Torr at 90%; 60 Torr at 93%; 80 Torr at 95%; and 100 Torr at 96% (4).

Distal diastolic pressure is more important than systolic pressure because the greatest proportion of flow occurs during diastole. Furthermore, endo perfusion probably occurs only during diastole (9). In this study, the critical diastolic pressure for the endo was 70 and for the epi 40 Torr. Below these respective values, regional Po_2 fell with further decreases in diastolic pressure.

Partial Release After Occlusion

Table 1 combines the results of two studies each on perfusion pressure changes and perfusion (H_2 clearance) and on perfusion pressure changes and Po_2. During the total occlusion, mean PCP was 20 and systolic/diastolic (S/D) PCP was

TABLE 1. *Occlusion, partial release, and total release*

	CBF[a] (% Cont.)[e]	PG[b] (mm Hg)	PCP[c] (mm Hg)	H_2C[d] (% Cont.)[e]		PO_2 (% Cont.)[e]	
				Epi	Endo	Epi	Endo
Basal	100	3.3	108 (119/97)[f]	100	100 1.13[g]	100	100 1.28[g]
Occlusion	0	88.7	20 (27/12)[f]	0	0	27	8 4.56[g]
Partial release	100	56.5	53 (73/33)[f]	92	0	106	25 9.56[g]
Total release	304	14.3	96 (110/81)[f]	165	275 0.67[g]	126	138 1.39[g]

[a] CBF, coronary blood flow by flowmeter.
[b] PG, pressure gradient.
[c] PCP, peripheral coronary pressure.
[d] H_2C—hydrogen clearance.
[e] % Cont.—percentage of control value.
[f] Systolic/diastolic pressure.
[g] Epi/endo ratio.

27/12 Torr, endo perfusion and epi perfusion were zero, and epi PO_2 and endo PO_2 were 27 and 8% of control values, respectively. Partial release to restore CBF to 100% control value permitted PCP S/D to return to 73/33 Torr. Epi perfusion returned to 92% of control, but endo perfusion remained at zero. Likewise, epi PO_2 returned to control, but endo remained depressed. Thus a diastolic pressure of 33 Torr was inadequate to restore endo perfusion. On total release, normal reactive hyperemia was observed in CBF and in epi and endo H_2 clearance; endo showed a greater percentage increase. The same was true for PO_2. Note that PCP was slightly below normal during RH, probably as a result of maximum vasodilatation. Furthermore, the pressure gradient was 14.3 compared to the control of 3.3. This was associated with the 300% increase in CBF.

DISCUSSION

Our studies show that the vasodilator autoregulatory reserve of the endo of the left ventricular free wall is considerably smaller than that of the epi. This difference in regional reserve becomes evident when CBF is increased in the presence of a critical stenosis of a large coronary artery. Thus, under basal conditions, transmural perfusion across the left ventricular wall is homogeneous, even in the presence of a "critical" stenosis; but when flow is elevated as a result of arteriolar dilatation distal to the stenosis, transmural perfusion becomes heterogeneous because of the greater increase in epi flow (1,4,7,13). In fact, under certain circumstances, endo flow may remain unchanged or actually decrease owing to a coronary "steal" phenomenon (1,11). It is essential that

CBF be elevated in order to measure coronary reserve and to demonstrate a regional perfusion deficit due to coronary stenosis (5,8). This is true in the clinical situation where the patient shows no sign of coronary insufficiency at rest, but will show such signs when the work load is increased and an imbalance between oxygen supply and demand develops in the endo. Therefore, during hyperemia resulting from an autoregulatory response to exercise, cardiac pacing, or a vasodilator agent, the effect of coronary stenosis can be seen as a perfusion imbalance.

The greater vulnerability of the endo to coronary stenosis is associated with a number of factors, including diastolic perfusion gradient, diastolic perfusion time, myocardial wall tension, and myocardial oxygen consumption (7,9). The deeper regions are perfused only during diastole, whereas the superficial epicardial vessels are perfused both during systole and diastole. Accordingly, there is a gradient of diastolic conductance with greater values for the endo region in order to maintain homogeneous average perfusion. Since the size of the arteriolar bed is probably the same throughout the left ventricular wall, there is a smaller arteriolar dilator reserve and a smaller capillary reserve under basal conditions (10,14). Oxygen utilization of the endo is greater than that of the epi. This explains the lower Po_2 since the supply of oxygen is similar in both regions but the requirement is greater in the endo (9,10). In the presence of a critical stenosis, homogeneous perfusion can be maintained at normal blood flow rates, but when blood flow is elevated, as during hyperemia, there is a pressure loss across the stenosis, producing a decrease in PCP distal to the stenosis. This then results in maldistribution of the blood flow since the perfusion pressure decreases with the increased blood flow and will be inadequate to perfuse the endo (1,7). The epi, with its greater arteriolar dilator reserve capacity, receives most of the blood flow and contributes to the decrease in the perfusion pressure. Under certain circumstances, perfusion pressure may be inadequate to maintain the patency of the endocardial arterioles, and in these instances critical closing occurs. This becomes particularly evident at maximum arteriolar dilatation in the presence of a flow restricting stenosis, such as demonstrated in the partial release experiments. Under those circumstances, perfusion of the endo did not recover (Figs. 8 and 9), whereas there was almost normal perfusion of the epi when blood flow was maintained at the control level. Thus all the flow went to the epi.

The vasodilator capacity of the arteriolar beds to maintain perfusion and normal blood flow distribution is great. Blood flow can increase as much as fourfold during maximal vasodilatation, as illustrated in Figs. 6 and 7. Diastolic perfusion pressure is well maintained in the presence of mild stenosis, and basal CBF will remain at normal levels with a stenosis of almost 90% (4). However, at the high flow rates, a 45% decrease in diameter, or about a 60 to 70% stenosis, will cause a diminution of the hyperemic response and an uneven distribution of flow. At that point, SR will become flow limiting. Our studies have demonstrated that endo reserve is exhausted at a diastolic pressure of 70 Torr and epi reserve at 40 Torr. These values are comparable to those of others

(7). When the regional reserve is exhausted, autoregulation can no longer compensate for the decrease in intraluminal pressure, and blood flow is directly related to perfusion pressure and ultimately to SR (11,16).

The changes in epi and endo Po_2 and perfusion with decreases in CBF demonstrate the linear relationship of endo Po_2 or perfusion to CBF when the reserve has been exhausted. This is well illustrated in Figs. 1 and 2. There were several steps of stenosis prior to the point of 0% change in mean CBF, but these were all less than critical. The epi curves demonstrate the autoregulatory compensatory reserve to maintain perfusion and Po_2, although not perfectly. But compensation fails and epi reserve is exhausted when mean CBF has been reduced about 70%; from that point on, the decline parallels that of endo. The overall pattern of change is better illustrated in Figs. 4 and 5. RH flow and overall coronary reserve (illustrated by the dark area) are gradually decreased. Endo reserve is exhausted when RH is reduced about 85% and basal CBF is diminished no more than 10%. All reserve is now in the epi region, and when this area becomes exhausted, RH is abolished and basal CBF is decreased 45 to 50%.

Acute occlusion of a coronary artery invariably leads to a more rapid decline in endo Po_2, which reaches a low level in a short period of time. Epi Po_2 declines more slowly and plateaus at a higher level. There are cases in which epi Po_2 may not decrease. Perfusion of both regions usually ceases on acute occlusion, but as in the case of the Po_2, there are times when epi perfusion will be maintained at a low level. Possibly this is due to the presence of interarterial anastomoses or collaterals to supply the epi. When the occlusion is released, reactive hyperemia occurs for mean CBF and regional perfusion as a result of maximal vasodilatation. The percentage increase may be greater in the endo region. The failure of regional Po_2 to overshoot is understandable in terms of oxygen balance. During the period of total occlusion, an oxygen debt was accumulated, and during the period of hyperemia, this is repaid to permit resynthesis of the metabolites required for myocardial contractility. As a result, Po_2 does not show an overshoot phenomenon.

Limiting reflow after transient acute occlusion points out some of the factors involved in maldistribution of blood flow. Po_2 and perfusion return almost to normal in the epi, but the endo remains unchanged. Thus the reflow is confined to the epi region. Perfusion pressure during the restricted reflow of partial release is 73/33 Torr, with a mean of 53 Torr. This is adequate to perfuse the epi, which receives blood flow during systole and diastole. The endo receives blood flow only during diastole, and the diastolic perfusion pressure of 33 Torr is not adequate. The wall tension is probably greater than that value (9). The critical closing pressure of the endo may be lower than that value, but it usually requires a greater pressure than the critical closing value to reopen an arteriolar bed (1). Other studies have demonstrated that the endo reserve is exhausted at the diastolic pressure of 70 Torr, and the pressure–flow relationship is linear from that point to about 30 Torr, when flow ceases. When pressure was reduced stepwise as illustrated in Fig. 10, CBF crossed the pressure axis at 13 to 20 Torr, which corresponds to critical closing pressure. Endo flow ceases at a higher value, possibly between 30 and 40 Torr, since the region is not perfused at 33 Torr. Epi critical closing is probably in the range of 15 to 20 Torr. One group suggested critical closing at 16 Torr (11); others propose a higher value of 20 to 54, with the endo at 32 and the epi at 17 Torr (9).

What is the clinical significance of the limited reflow studies? In the presence of a critical stenosis, coronary spasm followed by release would be similar to the acute occlusion and partial release. This situation would result in continued endo ischemia and could lead to infarction of that region, even though average CBF is normal. There is maldistribution of blood flow or coronary "steal" because the pressure distal to the stenosis is inadequate for perfusion of the endo region (1,4,11). When arteriolar tone is normal, epi "steal" will not occur and perfusion will be homogeneous.

REFERENCES

1. Bache, R. J., McHale, P. A., and Greenfield, J. C., Jr. (1977): Transmural myocardial perfusion during restricted coronary inflow in the awake dog. *Am. J. Physiol.,* 232:H645–H651.
2. Feldman, R. L., Nichols, W. W., Pepine, C. J., and Conti, C. R. (1978): Hemodynamic significance of the length of a coronary arterial narrowing. *Am. J. Cardiol.,* 41:865–871.
3. Gould, K. L., and Lipscomb, K. (1974): Effects of coronary stenosis on coronary flow reserve and resistance. *Am. J. Cardiol.,* 34:48–55.
4. Gould, K. L., Lipscomb, K., and Calvert, C. (1975): Compensatory changes of the distal coronary vascular bed during progressive coronary constriction. *Circulation,* 51:1083–1094.
5. Gould, K. L., Lipscomb, K., and Hamilton, G. W. (1974): Physiologic basis for assessing critical coronary stenosis: Instantaneous flow response and regional distribution during coronary hyperemia as measures of coronary flow reserve. *Am. J. Cardiol.,* 33:87–94.
6. Gross, G. J., and Winbury, M. M. (1973): Beta adrenergic blockade on intramyocardial distribution of coronary blood flow. *J. Pharmacol. Exp. Ther.,* 187:451–464.
7. Guyton, R. A., McClenathan, J. H., Newman, G. E., and Michaelis, L. L. (1977): Significance of subendocardial S-T segment elevation caused by coronary stenosis in the dog: Epicardial S-T segment depression, local ischemia, and subsequent necrosis. *Am. J. Cardiol.,* 40:373–380.
8. Hillis, W. S., and Friesinger, G. C. (1976): Reactive hyperemia: An index of the significance of coronary stenosis. *Am. Heart J.,* 92:737–740.
9. Hoffman, J. I. E. (1978): Determinants and prediction of transmural myocardial perfusion. *Circulation,* 58:381–391.
10. Howe, B. B., Weiss, H. R., Wilkes, S. B., and Winbury, M. M. (1975): Pentaerythritol trinitrate and glyceryl trinitrate on intramyocardial oxygenation and perfusion in the dog. Krogh analysis of transmural metabolism. *Clin. Exp. Pharmacol. Physiol.,* 2:529–540.
11. Lipscomb, K., and Gould, K. L. (1975): Mechanism of the effect of coronary artery stenosis on coronary flow in the dog. *Am. Heart J.,* 89:60–67.
12. Mates, R. E., Gupta, R. L., Bell, A. C., and Klocke, F. J. (1978): Fluid dynamics of coronary artery stenosis. *Circ. Res.,* 42:152–162.
13. Nakamura, M., Matsuguchi, H., Mitsutake, A., Kikuchi, Y., Takeshita, A., Nakagaki, O., and Kuroiwa, A. (1977): The effect of graded coronary stenosis on myocardial blood flow and left ventricular wall motion. *Basic Res. Cardiol.,* 72:479–491.
14. Winbury, M. M., Howe, B. B., and Weiss, H. R. (1971): Effect of nitroglycerin and dipyridamole on epicardial and endocardial oxygen tension—Further evidence for redistribution of myocardial blood flow. *J. Pharmacol. Exp. Ther.,* 176:184—199.
15. Yokoyama, M., Maekawa, K., Katada, Y., Ishikawa, Y., Azumi, T., Mizutani, T., Fukuzaki, H., and Tomomatsu, T. (1978): Effects of graded coronary constriction on regional oxygen and carbon dioxide tensions in outer and inner layers of the canine myocardium. *Jpn. Circ. J.,* 42:701–709.
16. Young, D. F., Cholvin, N. R., Kirkeeide, R. L., and Roth, A. C. (1977): Hemodynamics of arterial stenosis at elevated flow rates. *Circ. Res.,* 41:99–107.

Ischemic Myocardium and Antianginal Drugs,
edited by M. M. Winbury and Y. Abiko.
Raven Press, New York © 1979.

Ca^{2+} Antagonism in Various Parameters of Cardiac Function Including Coronary Dilatation with the Use of Nifedipine, Perhexiline, and Verapamil

Hiroshi Ono and Koroku Hashimoto

Hatano Research Institute, Food and Drug Safety Center, Kanagawa 257, Japan

Although some of the metal ions have been discovered to block competitively calcium influx through the myocardial membrane (7), their use in the physiological study of the role of calcium ion in excitation–contraction coupling has been limited. Recently some organic compounds with highly specific Ca^{2+} antagonistic activity—verapamil, D$_{600}$, prenylamine (8), and nifedipine (4,5)—have been synthesized and studied extensively. Their essential pharmacological property as coronary vasodilators has been ascribed to the inhibition of Ca^{2+} influx into the vascular smooth muscle cell. In addition, the energy conserving property of these compounds on the myocardium has been found to be useful for the treatment of ischemic heart disorder, especially in reducing mechanical or metabolic hyperactivity. The number of publications on the role of Ca^{2+} in biological, biochemical, and physiological phenomena is growing rapidly. Enzyme reactions, endocrine and exocrine secretion, exocytosis of catecholamine granules at the nerve terminal, movement of spermatozoa, and other activities are all inhibited by Ca^{2+} antagonists but to different degrees. Thus it is important to clarify the differences in sensitivity to Ca^{2+} antagonists, especially for mutually related parameters such as cardiac function and coronary vascular tone, in order to evaluate their therapeutic usefulness.

In this chapter, we present the recent results concerning the effects of nifedipine, perhexiline, and verapamil on blood-perfused excised canine myocardial preparations compared with systemic responses in dogs.

METHODS

Our methods entailed use of excised canine myocardial preparations perfused with blood of a donor dog and have been developed and used extensively by our colleagues and by us. The heart of a dog was excised under pentobarbital anesthesia and immediately plunged in chilled Tyrode solution at 15°C. The sinoatrial node–right atrial preparation (1) and the papillary muscle preparation

(2) were made as follows (since details are described in the references cited above, only a brief outline is given). The sinoatrial node and the surrounding right atrial free wall were perfused with blood through the cannulated sinus-node artery. The ventricular border of the right atrium was fixed on a steel plate, and the tension development was measured isometrically with a force-displacement transducer (Grass FT03). Sinus rate was measured continuously by a cardiotachograph (Datagraph T419) triggered by the atrial electrogram. For the papillary muscle preparation, the anterior septal branch of the anterior descending artery was cannulated, and the developed tension of the anterior papillary muscle of the right ventricle driven at the rate of 120/min was measured isometrically. Both preparations were set in a water jacket warmed to 37°C and perfused with blood from the carotid artery of a donor dog at constant pressure of 80 mm Hg, using a perfusion pump (Harvard 1215) and a pneumatic resistance. The blood flow rate through the papillary muscle preparation was measured with an electromagnetic flowmeter (Narco RT500). The venous out-flow of the preparations was returned to the jugular vein of the donor dog (Fig. 1). A donor dog was anesthetized with pentobarbital sodium, and coagula-tion was prevented with heparin sodium (Sigma). Systemic blood pressure of the donor was measured at the femoral artery by a Statham transducer (P 23Db) and heart rate with another tachograph triggered by the blood pressure pulses. In some experiments, the thorax was opened at the right third intercostal space under artificial respiration, and a Morawitz cannula was inserted into the coronary sinus through an incision at the apex of the right auricle. Coronary outflow was led to an extracorporeal circuit between the coronary sinus and

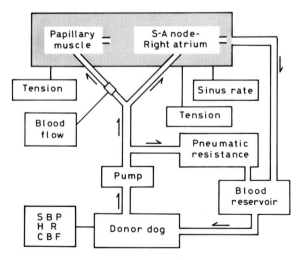

FIG. 1. Diagram of the experimental arrangement. SBP, systemic blood flow; CSF, coronary sinus blood flow.

the jugular vein. An electromagnetic flowmeter probe was interposed in the extracorporeal circuit to measure the coronary sinus outflow.

In another series of experiments, various vascular beds were perfused and their responses to the drugs were studied. The left femoral artery, the circumflex branch of the left coronary artery, the left renal artery, or the superior mesenteric artery was cannulated and perfused at a constant pressure of 100 mm Hg with heparinized blood pumped from the right femoral artery. Responses of the vascular beds were studied with an electromagnetic flowmeter.

Nifedipine (Bayer) was a solution in an organic solvent provided by the manufacturer; perhexiline hydrochloride (Merrell) was dissolved in distilled water; and verapamil hydrochloride (Eisai) was dissolved in 0.9% saline. Since the concentration of the solution of perhexiline was limited (0.2%), the injection was performed slowly to avoid volume effect. Doses of the drugs were expressed as their bases.

RESULTS

Effects of Verapamil, Nifedipine, and Perhexiline on Blood-Perfused Preparations of the Canine Right Atrium

Test drugs were injected intra-arterially, close to the preparations. Verapamil—the most frequently studied Ca^{2+} antagonist in the cardiohemodynamic study (9)—induced dose-related decreases of both sinus rate and right atrial contraction and finally induced sinus arrest (Fig. 2). Responses to nifedipine

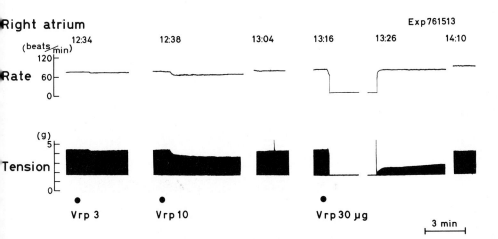

FIG. 2. Effect of verapamil (Vrp) on the excised blood-perfused right atrial preparation of a dog. Verapamil (30 μg i.a.) induced sinus arrest followed by spontaneous recovery to the normal rate after 10 min; contractile force recovered gradually over a long period.

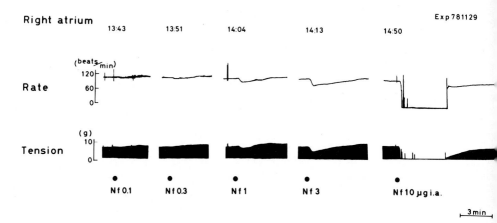

FIG. 3. Effect of nifedipine (Nf) on the excised blood-perfused right atrial preparation of a dog. Sinus rate recovered within 5 min from the arrest induced by 10 μg of nifedipine.

were quite similar to those to verapamil, but its potency was a little greater (Fig. 3). Perhexiline—a recently developed coronary vasodilator that is reported to be useful, especially for the treatment of angina of effort (12)—showed similar responses to verapamil, but its potency was 10 times less than that of verapamil on the weight basis. A slight positive inotropic effect was observed following an initial negative one at a lower dose level. With increasing doses, sinus arrest occurred after a marked decrease of the sinus rate (Fig. 4).

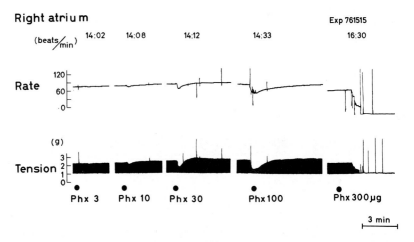

FIG. 4. Effect of perhexiline (Phx) on the excised blood-perfused right atrial preparation of a dog. Sinus rate had not recovered at 30 min from the sinus arrest induced by 300 μg of perhexiline.

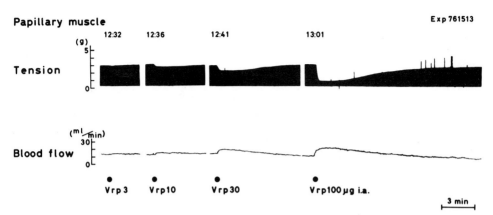

FIG. 5. Effect of verapamil (Vrp) on the excised blood-perfused papillary muscle preparation of a dog, measuring tension and blood flow. Muscle was driven at 120/min.

Effects of Verapamil, Nifedipine, and Perhexiline on Blood-Perfused Papillary Muscle Preparations

Test drugs were given intra-arterially, close to the preparations. Verapamil induced a dose-related depression of papillary muscle contraction with a simultaneous increase of blood flow of the nourishing artery (Fig. 5). Nifedipine had similar effects, but was about 10 times more potent than verapamil for inducing the vasodilator effect (Fig. 6). Perhexiline showed an initial negative and a subsequent slight positive inotropic effect together with a vasodilator effect. The positive inotropic effect produced by perhexiline was slight but definite

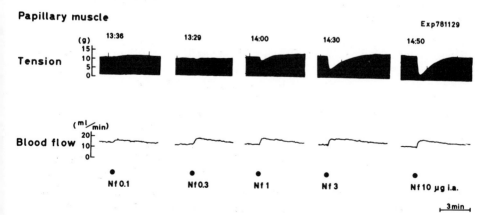

FIG. 6. Effect of nifedipine (Nf) on the excised blood-perfused papillary muscle preparation of a dog, measuring tension and blood flow.

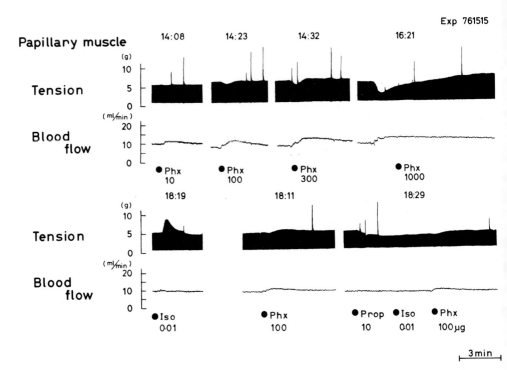

FIG. 7. Effect of perhexiline (Phx) on the excised, blood-perfused papillary muscle preparation of a dog. A slight positive inotropic effect induced with 100 μg perhexiline was not blocked by treatment with 10 μg propranolol (Prop), which completely blocked the positive inotropic effect of 0.01 μg isoproterenol (Iso).

and could not be inhibited by treatment with propranolol (Fig. 7). Potencies of perhexiline were 10 times less than verapamil in both the vasodilator and the inotropic effects.

Simultaneous Observation of Effects of Verapamil, Perhexiline, and Nifedipine on Systemic Blood Pressure and Heart Rate and on Blood-Perfused Preparations of Right Atrium and Papillary Muscle

Test drugs were given intravenously to the donor dog. Verapamil and perhexiline induced dose-related decreases in systemic blood pressure and heart rate, but reflex tachycardia occasionally made the responses more complex. Dose-related increases in coronary flow paralleled the changes in blood pressure and heart rate. When a large dose of verapamil (300 μg/kg) was injected, the sinus rhythm and the atrioventricular conduction were so impaired that arrhythmias occurred frequently (Fig. 8). Thus the increased coronary blood flow was influenced by an arrhythmic slow ventricular rate. The vasodilator responses that were observed in both the coronary sinus outflow and the nourishing artery

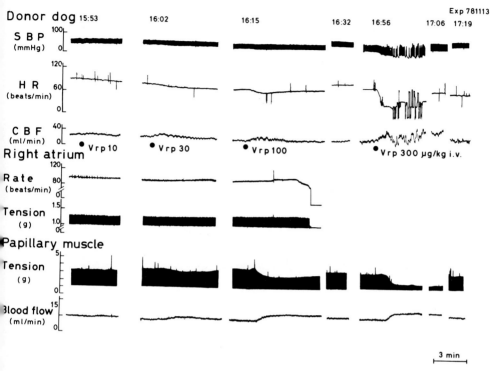

FIG. 8. Effect of verapamil (Vrp) on an open-chest dog and the excised preparations perfused with the blood of this dog. SBP, systemic blood pressure; HR, heart rate; and CBF, coronary blood flow of the donor dog. Rate and tension of the right atrium and tension and blood flow of the papillary muscle were simultaneously observed.

of the papillary muscle preparation were more evident than other parameters of cardiac function, and the sinus arrest of the right atrial preparation occurred earlier than others. Perhexiline induced sinus arrest and positive and negative inotropic effects in the excised blood-perfused preparations but never induced second-degree atrioventricular block, even with the highest hypotensive dose (10 mg/kg). The initial increase in the coronary sinus outflow was modified by the maximal hypotensive effect with 10 mg/kg, but a gradual increase in a later phase reached almost the same level of the initial increase, as shown in Fig. 9. Nifedipine—the most potent Ca²⁺ antagonist—induced a remarkable increase in coronary flow, even when cardiac function was slightly affected. As in the case of perhexiline, severe block of the atrioventricular conduction did not occur *in vivo*, even when the maximal hypotensive response modified the coronary blood flow. The nifedipine-induced coronary dilatation lasted considerably longer than that induced by the other agents (Fig. 10).

In the case of verapamil, the negative inotropic effect on the blood-perfused papillary muscle preparation was quite parallel with the changes in systemic

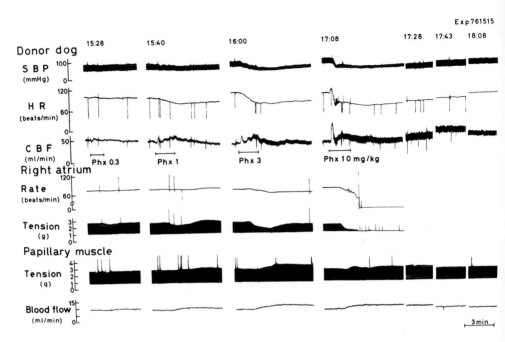

FIG. 9. Effect of perhexiline (Phx) on an open-chest dog and excised preparations perfused with blood of this dog. SBP, systemic blood pressure; HR, heart rate; and CBF, coronary blood flow of the donor dog. Rate and tension of the right atrium and tension and blood flow of the papillary muscle were simultaneously observed.

blood pressure, heart rate, coronary blood flow *in vivo,* and blood flow in the nourishing vessel of the anterior septal artery. The perhexiline-induced negative inotropic response, however, was followed by a positive one. Nifedipine induced a dose-related negative inotropic effect that was, however, slight and short lasting.

Comparison of Vascular Responses Among Various Vascular Beds

Responses to verapamil and perhexiline were examined in this study. The femoral arterial bed showed the greatest relative response followed closely by the coronary vascular bed; the renal and mesenteric beds had smaller responses to either verapamil or perhexiline. However, there are some differences between verapamil and perhexiline. The renal artery responded frequently in different patterns, such as vasoconstriction with perhexiline, even when the perfusion pressure was controlled at the constant level. The coronary artery responded about the same as the femoral with verapamil, while it responded less than the femoral artery with perhexiline (Figs. 11 and 12). The responses of the mesenteric artery were only examined with perhexiline and were between those of the renal and the coronary arteries (Fig. 12).

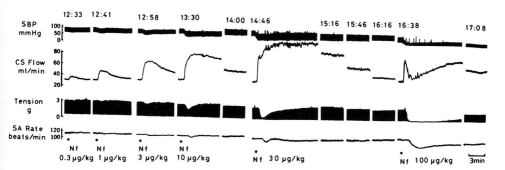

FIG. 10. Effect of nifedipine on an open-chest dog and the excised preparations perfused with the blood of this dog. SBP, systemic blood pressure and CS flow, coronary sinus blood flow of the donor dog. Tension of the papillary muscle and sinoatrial (SA) rate of the excised preparations were simultaneously observed.

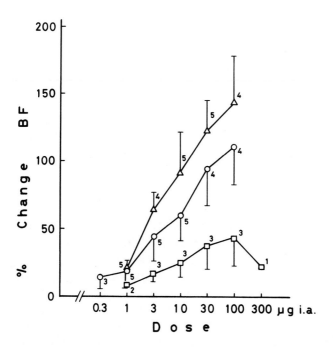

FIG. 11. Effect of verapamil on the blood flow (BF) rate of the coronary *(circles)*, femoral *(triangles)*, and renal *(squares)* arteries. Numbers near the symbols indicate the number of observations. The effects on various arteries are expressed in percentage change.

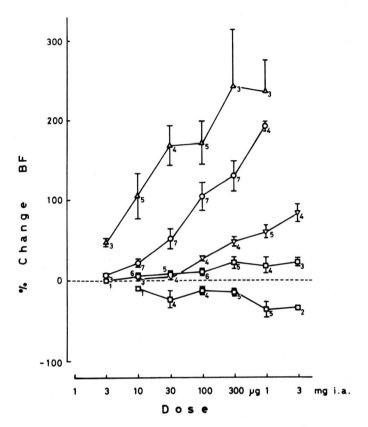

FIG. 12. Effect of perhexiline on the blood flow (BF) rate of the coronary *(circles)*, femoral *(triangles)*, mesenteric *(inverted triangles)*, and renal *(squares)* arteries. Numbers near the symbols indicate the number of observations.

DISCUSSION

As parameters of cardiac function, papillary muscle contraction (6), sinoatrial rate (11), and atrioventricular conduction (10) were precisely analyzed with excised blood-perfused preparations. The dose–response relations of verapamil, nifedipine, diltiazem, and other drugs were compared with respect to negative inotropic, chronotropic, and dromotropic effects, together with the vasodilator effect on the nourishing arteries. Potencies for decreasing sinus rate and atrioventricular conduction were almost the same for verapamil and nifedipine, but for depression of the papillary muscle contraction and vasodilatation, nifedipine was 10 times more potent than verapamil, as shown in Table 1. Thus direct effects on papillary muscle contraction and coronary vascular tone were more Ca^{2+} dependent than those on sinus automaticity and atrioventricular conduction. Recently, Endoh et al. (3) reported that automaticity of Purkinje fibers

TABLE 1. *Relative potencies of Ca²⁺-antagonistic vasodilators on various cardiovascular functions*[a]

	Nifedipine	Verapamil	Diltiazem	Perhexiline[e]
Negative chronotropic action[b]	1	1	1/3	(1/30)
Negative inotropic action[c]	1	1/13	1/40	(1/100)
Negative dromotropic action[d]	1	1/2	1/2	(1/100)
Vasodilator action[c]	1	1/12	1/26	(1/36)

[a]Determined with the excised blood-perfused myocardial preparations of the dog.
[b]On the sinoatrial node preparation [from Ono et al. (11)].
[c]On the papillary muscle preparation [from Himori et al. (6)].
[d]On the atrioventricular node preparation [from Narimatsu and Taira (10)].
[e]Approximate values; obtained with the same methods in a different study (Ono, O'Hara, Oguro, and Hashimoto, *unpublished data*).

was depressed by the calcium ion in contrast to the sinoatrial node and that it was quite resistant to Ca²⁺ antagonists (i.e., almost no response to nifedipine but slight dual response to verapamil). Thus even among cardiac functions, there are significant differences in the degree of calcium dependency.

In the whole animal, coronary vasodilatation was considerably more sensitive than any other cardiac parameter to nifedipine, whereas with verapamil, vasodilatation and the negative inotropic response occurred at similar doses, as demonstrated in this study. Previously, Kokubun ct al. (9) compared the cardiohemodynamic effects of various vasodilators and showed that nifedipine induced a definite increase of cardiac output. On the other hand, verapamil produced a decrease of cardiac output and an increase of right atrial pressure, even though the venous return was reduced; this indicates a depression of the cardiac function by verapamil. On the contrary, nifedipine increased cardiac output and venous return and also right atrial pressure. Perhexiline increased, though slightly, both cardiac output and venous return (H. Ono and K. Hashimoto, *unpublished observation*). Perhexiline was also different from verapamil in that no depression of atrioventricular conduction was observed within a dose range for vasodilator effect.

Among Ca²⁺ antagonists, cardiovascular responses showed such wide differences that it is important to examine the whole pharmacological profile (including other associated properties) of these drugs in order to evaluate correctly their clinical usefulness for various types of disease. It is important to note the following from these studies: (a) Ca²⁺-dependent phenomena, even among cardiac functions, show various sensitivities to Ca²⁺ antagonists. (b) An erroneous conclusion will be drawn by combining the results of various dose–response relations obtained from a variety of preparations, without considering the differences in importance of the calcium ion in various calcium-dependent biological phenomena.

REFERENCES

1. Chiba, S., Kimura, T., and Hashimoto, K. (1975): Muscarinic suppression of the nicotinic action of acetylcholine on the isolated, blood-perfused atrium of the dog. *Naunyn Schmiedebergs Arch. Pharmacol.,* 289:315–325.
2. Endoh, M., and Hashimoto, K. (1970): Pharmacological evidence of autonomic nerve activities in canine papillary muscle. *Am. J. Physiol.,* 218:1459–1463.
3. Endoh, M., Yanagisawa, T., and Taira, N. (1978): Effects of calcium-antagonistic coronary vasodilators, nifedipine and verapamil, on ventricular automaticity of the dog. *Naunyn Schmiedebergs Arch. Pharmacol.,* 302:235–238.
4. Fleckenstein, A., Tritthart, H., Döring, H.-J., and Byon, K. Y. (1972): BAYa1040–ein hochaktiver Ca⁺⁺-antagonistischer Inhibitor der elecktromechanischer Kopplungsprozesse ein Warmblüter-Myokard. *Arzneim. Forsch.,* 22:22–33.
5. Hashimoto, K., Taira, N., Chiba, S., Hashimoto, K., Jr., Endoh, M., Kokubun, M., Kokubun, H., Iijima, T., Kimura, T., Kubota, K., and Oguro, K. (1972): Cardiohemodynamic effects of BAYa1040 in the dog. *Arzneim. Forsch.,* 22:15–21.
6. Himori, N., Ono, H., and Taira, N. (1976): Simultaneous assessment of effects of coronary vasodilators on the coronary blood flow and the myocardial contractility by using the blood-perfused canine papillary muscle. *Jpn. J. Pharmacol.,* 26:427–435.
7. Kaufmann, R., and Fleckenstein, A. (1965): Ca⁺⁺-kompetitive elektro-mechanische Entkopplung durch Ni⁺⁺- und Co⁺⁺-Ionen am Warmblütermyokard. *Pfluegers Arch.,* 282:290–297.
8. Kohlhardt, M., Bauer, B., Krause, H., and Fleckenstein, A. (1972): Differentiation of the transmembrane Na and Ca channels in mammalian cardiac fibres by the use of specific inhibitors. *Pfluegers Arch.,* 335:309–322.
9. Kokubun, M., Taira, N., and Hashimoto, K. (1974): Cardiohemodynamic effects of nitroglycerin and several vasodilators. *Jpn. Heart J.,* 15:126–144.
10. Narimatsu, A., and Taira, N. (1976): Effects on atrio-ventricular conduction of calcium-antagonistic coronary vasodilators, local anesthetics and quinidine injected into the posterior and the anterior septal artery of the atrio-ventricular node preparation of the dog. *Naunyn Schmiedebergs Arch. Pharmacol.,* 294:169–177.
11. Ono, H., Himori, N., and Taira, N. (1977): Chronotropic effects of coronary vasodilators as assessed in the isolated, blood-perfused sino-atrial preparation of the dog. *Tohoku J. Exp. Med.,* 121:383–390.
12. *Perhexiline Maleate. Proceedings of a Symposium,* edited by A. Fleckenstein, W. Klaus, A. A. Sunahara, G. A. Neuhaus, and A. Perrin. Excerpta Medica, Amsterdam (1978).

Ischemic Myocardium and Antianginal Drugs,
edited by M. M. Winbury and Y. Abiko.
Raven Press, New York © 1979.

Mechanisms of Antianginal Drugs

*Richard J. Bing, Ronald Weishaar, Angelika Rackl,
and Günter Pawlik

*Huntington Institute of Applied Medical Research and the Huntington Memorial Hospital,
Pasadena, California 91105; and *University of Southern California, Los Angeles,
California 90023, and California Institute of Technology, Pasadena, California 91109*

Antianginal agents have been used since Brunton (6) first described the effect of amyl nitrate and related it to a fall in arterial blood pressure due to vasodilatation of the systemic vessels. Since then, a variety of drugs have been employed for the treatment of angina pectoris. Most of the studies carried out within the last two decades have dealt with problems related to myocardial infarction rather than angina pectoris. Only a few studies have dealt with the circulatory changes in heart muscle and systemic circulation (2,4,11).

The purpose of this chapter is to review the circulatory effects and the action on cardiac metabolism of antianginal drugs. The first section deals with an overview of the action of antianginal drugs on cardiac metabolism and circulatory changes. The second is concerned with the action of the calcium antagonist diltiazem on regional myocardial ischemia before and after the resumption of coronary flow.

ACTION OF ANTIANGINAL DRUGS

Anginal drugs can be divided into three major groups: those with an action that is primarily hemodynamic (redistribution of blood flow in the systemic and coronary circulation); beta blockers; and calcium antagonists. No mention will be made here of drugs that alter pre- or afterload or that, by other mechanisms, reduce the size of a myocardial infarct. The action of Intensain® (chromonar) will not be discussed here since it has been extensively reviewed in previous publications (3).

Drugs That Act Primarily on the Hemodynamics

Nitrites are the prototypes of this group. Within recent years, another preparation—molsidomin—has appeared with similar action (34). No definite action of these drugs on cardiac metabolism has been demonstrated, although Ogawa et al. (29) discovered a monoamine oxidase inhibitory effect of nitroglycerin on the heart. Early reports postulated that nitroglycerin exerts its action primarily through coronary vasodilatation (10,26). An often forgotten fact is that nitroglycerin does not increase *total* coronary blood flow in the presence of coronary arteriosclerosis (7). Nitroglycerin causes a redistribution of regional myocardial blood flow after ischemia (2). Cohen et al. (8) have shown that nitrites can dilate collateral vessels. Using xenon, Horwitz et al. (17) demonstrated that nitroglycerin improved perfusion in regions of diseased myocardium in patients with coronary artery disease.

Of importance is the effect of nitroglycerin on peripheral circulation. Williams et al. (40) discovered that, possibly as a result of peripheral vasodilatation and pooling, ventricular size and intraventricular systolic pressure diminished and that both end-diastolic and end-systolic ventricular dimensions decreased. Since these factors determine the degree of myocardial wall tension, and since ventricular tension is an important determinant of myocardial oxygen consumption, a decline in myocardial tension results in a diminution in myocardial oxygen demands.

The effect of nitrites on the systemic venous bed, particularly systemic vascular volume and venous distensibility, has brought to the foreground the importance of this portion of the circulation in the action of antianginal agents (32). For example, the systemic venous bed responds to stimulation of venous alpha and beta receptors by vasoconstriction and thus increases venous return and cardiac output (24).

In many respects, molsidomin—a new antianginal agent—acts similarly to nitroglycerin, that is, primarily on the capacity and compliance of the systemic venous system. However, in contrast to nitroglycerin, its action is more prolonged. Schartl et al. (34) employed venous occlusion plethysmography and found a left shift of the pressure–volume curve in the veins of the human forearm. At identical intravenous pressure, the drug resulted in a disproportionate increase in volume; in other words, the capacity of the venous bed increased and venous return to the heart diminished. They also showed by scintigraphic measurements a diminution of the percentage of total blood volume in the thorax, with an increase in the abdomen. In another study, no metabolic changes in heart muscle following the administration of molsidomin were found (R. Weishaar and R. J. Bing, *unpublished observations*).

Beta Blockers

In 1948, Ahlquist (1) introduced the concept of a dual alpha- and beta-adrenergic receptor mechanism to explain contrasting responses to various amines. In 1964, Black et al. (5) described an antagonist of isoproterenol—propranolol. In 1964 and 1965, the usefulness of propranolol in the treatment of angina pectoris was reported (13,37). In 1967, Robin et al. (31), using a specially designed strain gauge catheter, found that, like nitroglycerin, propranolol resulted in a decrease in shortening of human heart muscle *in vivo*. There was, however, one significant difference: Propranolol caused a marked increase in left ventricular end-diastolic pressure. Therefore, this beta blocker had a direct effect on cardiac contractility.

Other effects of propranolol were soon published. Kloner et al. (22) in 1976 found that propranolol decreased the absolute flow to both the inner and outer halves of ischemic myocardium without significant change in the endo-/epicardial flow ratio. Therefore, the drug does not improve the perfusion to the ischemic myocardium.

It is, therefore, likely that propranolol has antianginal properties because—as shown by Nayler et al. (27), Robin and Bing (31), and Gross and Winbury (14)—it diminishes myocardial oxygen demands and coronary flow. It does this by affecting two determinants of myocardial oxygen demands—myocardial contractility and heart rate. It also decreases, particularly in hypertensive individuals, the blood pressure.

Propranolol also appears to have a direct effect on myocardial substrate metabolism. Marchetti et al. (23) found that beta blockers decrease myocardial extraction of fatty acids. Opie and Thomas (30) described that the drug increased myocardial glucose extraction and diminished myocardial extraction of fatty acids. Free fatty acid content in ischemic heart muscle diminished. Weishaar and Bing (38) have recently shown an increase in fatty acids in the ischemic region of the myocardium. Whether the action of propranolol results from increased mitochondrial oxidation of fatty acids or from increased activity of palmitoyl-CoA synthetase or carnitine palmitoyl transferase has not been established. In any case, beta blockade may alter metabolic pathways in the heart muscle. This also has been found in man by Mueller et al. (25).

Calcium Antagonists

Calcium ions are the link between excitation and contraction. The chain of events begins at the sarcolemma; then calcium passes through the T system of the sarcoplasmic reticulum and to the contractile elements. The sarcolemma is a complicated structure consisting of, among other components, a surface coat that is of importance in Ca^{2+} transfer (9). The action potential is composed of several phases: depolarization, the plateau, and repolarization. The ion movements that affect depolarization and repolarization are electrogenic in that they give rise to electrical currents (20). During depolarization, Na^+ moves inward; during early repolarization, K^+ moves outward. The plateau phase is dominated by the slow inward current that is carried by calcium. It is this slow phase of the action potential that is blocked by calcium antagonists (12). The pronounced negative inotropic effect of these drugs is the result of this blockage of Ca^{2+} across the sarcolemma. These compounds selectively abolish the contractile response of isolated papillary muscle without any change in action potential (12). Therefore, they block contraction but do not interfere with Na^+ movement across the sarcolemma, which occurs during the fast phase of the action potential.

Because of the negative inotropic effects of these drugs, less ATP is consumed, and ATP in fact accumulates in the myocardium. A consequence of the decrease in high-energy phosphate consumption is that the calcium antagonists also reduce the cardiac oxygen requirements (12). Obviously, these factors form the basis of the antianginal effects of these drugs and for the protection of the ischemic and the ischemic–reperfused myocardium.

EFFECT OF DILTIAZEM ON ISCHEMIC AND ISCHEMIC–REPERFUSED MYOCARDIUM

The biochemical changes during myocardial ischemia affect, among other things, mitochondrial respiration, calcium uptake and binding by mitochondria and by sarcoplasmic reticulum and glycolytic pathway intermediates, free fatty acids, and high-energy phosphates. As a result of these changes, myocardial contractility is reduced. Weishaar and Bing (39) showed that 1 to 3 hr after the onset of ischemia, mitochondrial respiration, particularly mitochondrial oxygen consumption, was depressed. Schwartz et al. (35) demonstrated a depression of state 3 respiration. They also found diminished mitochondrial Ca^{2+} uptake with subsequent release of the calcium taken up by the mitochondria during continued respiratory activity. Marked impairment of Ca^{2+} binding and release from sarcoplasmic reticulum of ischemic myocardium was also present. Myocardial ischemia also blocks the activity of rate-limiting enzymes, such as phosphofructokinase (PFK) and glyceraldehyde-3-phosphate dehydrogenase (G-3-PDH) (28,39). Therefore, ischemia inhibits total flux through the glycolytic pathway. Decline in high-energy phosphates has also been demonstrated (39). As a result of these changes, myocardial contractility is reduced, as illustrated in glycerinated heart muscle from ischemic tissue (39).

In the experiments reported here, it could be shown that the calcium antagonist diltiazem effectively counteracts some of the effects of acute myocardial ischemia. The experiments were carried out on dogs with myocardial ischemia initiated by ligating several smaller branches of the left anterior descending coronary artery. The extent of heart muscle affected by ischemia was estimated by the injection of 10% alphazurine 2G blue dye 5 min prior to sacrifice, as described by Kane et al. (19). This dye stains only well-perfused tissue and permits demarcation of the ischemic regions. Two groups of dogs were examined: In the first, no medication was given during the ischemic period; in the second, diltiazem hydrochloride (0.2 mg/kg dissolved in sterile saline) was administered as a bolus injection 10 min after ligation. All animals were sacrificed after 60 min of ischemia. Immediately prior to sacrifice, tissue samples were removed for determination of glycolytic intermediates and high-energy phosphates. Samples for determination of regional coronary blood flow and free fatty acids and for studies of contractility of glycerinated muscle fibers and isolation of mitochondria were then collected following removal of the heart.

The following glycolytic intermediates were measured: lactate, pyruvate, α-glycerophosphate (α-GP), dihydroxyacetone phosphate (DHAP), glucose-6-phosphate (G-6-P), fructose-6-phosphate (F-6-P), and fructose 1,6-diphosphate (F-1,6-DP). The myocardial redox state was monitored by comparing the ratio of lactate to pyruvate and of α-GP to DHAP. In addition, glycolytic flux through PFK, a key regulatory enzyme for anaerobic glycolysis, was estimated using the formula

$$\text{Glycolytic flux} = (G\text{-}6\text{-}P) + (F\text{-}6\text{-}P)/(F\text{-}1,6\text{-}DP).$$

Tissue levels of high-energy phosphates—creatine phosphate (CP), adenosine-5'-triphosphate (ATP), and adenosine-5'-diphosphate (ADP)—were also measured. The tissue levels of the following free fatty acids were determined: myristic, palmitic, stearic, oleic, and linoleic acids. Contractility of glycerinated heart muscle fibers was measured according to methods described from this laboratory (33). Measurements were carried out in a servo system that maintained constant length while increasing tension was recorded. From the data obtained during this isometric contraction, the following indices could be determined: maximal developed tension (P_o), time to peak tension (t_o), and the maximal rate of tension development (dp/dt_{max}).

Mitochondrial respiration was measured with a Gilson oxygraph using, in principle, a method of Schwartz (35), and mitochondrial calcium binding was measured according to the millipore filter method of Harigaya and Schwartz (15).

Administration of diltiazem lessened the effect of ischemia in several ways (Table 1). While ATP levels were reduced by roughly 50% of the nonischemic value in the control group, this reduction was only about 25% in the diltiazem-treated dogs (Fig. 1). This represents a marked preservation of the energy reservoir in these animals. In addition, the fall in ADP in the ischemic region was prevented by the administration of diltiazem.

The level of lactate in the ischemic tissue was considerably lower in the diltiazem-treated dogs than in the control animals (Fig. 2). In addition to lactate,

TABLE 1. *Effects of diltiazem on biochemical processes in ischemic heart muscle*

1. ATP preserved, fall in ADP prevented[a]
2. t_o diminished, P_o increased, dp/dt_{max} increased[b]
3. Glycolytic flux increased
4. FFA and lactate lower[c]
5. Mitochondrial respiration unchanged

[a] ATP, adenosine-5'-triphosphate; ADP, adenosine-5'-diphosphate.

[b] t_o, time to peak tension; P_o, maximal tension developed; dp/dt_{max}, maximal rate of tension development.

[c] FFA, free fatty acid.

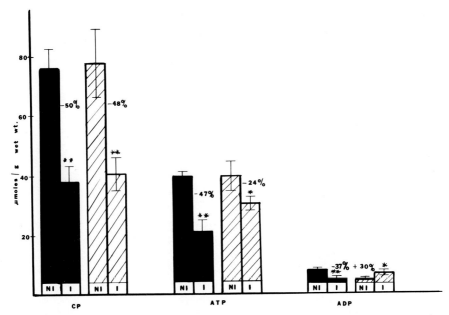

FIG. 1. The effect of diltiazem on high-energy phosphate levels in ischemic (I) heart muscle. The drug lessens the fall in ATP and ADP. NI, nonischemic; *solid bars,* control (no drug); *slashed bars,* diltiazem; *, $0.05 < p < 0.10$; **, $p < 0.05$.

the level of α-GP in the occluded region did not rise as high as that in the ischemic tissue taken from the dogs not given diltiazem. Free fatty acid (FFA) concentration in heart muscle was lower in animals treated with diltiazem in both ischemic and nonischemic regions (Fig. 3).

Figure 2 shows also that ischemia produced a 3.9-fold increase in the lactate/pyruvate ratio in the control animals and a 3.3-fold rise in the α-GP/DHAP ratio. Administration of diltiazem lessened to a slight degree the effect of ischemia on the lactate/pyruvate ratio but had no effect on the rise in the α-GP/DHAP ratio in the occluded region. As shown in Fig. 4, the levels of both G-6-P and F-6-P increased sharply with ischemia in the control group. At the same time, F-1,6-DP levels declined, indicating inhibition of PFK. In dogs receiving diltiazem, the elevations in G-6-P and F-6-P were about the same as in the animals not receiving the drug, but the fall in F-1,6-DP was not as large. As a result of these changes, there was a 2.8-fold inhibition of the glycolytic flux in the control dogs and only a 1.6-fold inhibition in the diltiazem-treated animals, indicating that the inhibition of glycolytic flux at the PFK level was lessened by diltiazem administration (Fig. 4).

Studies of *in vitro* contractility using glycerinated heart muscle fibers demonstrated that diltiazem administration led to a marked reduction in ischemia-induced damage to the contractile elements (Fig. 5). In the animals not receiving diltiazem, values for P_o and dp/dt_{max} were reduced in ischemic muscle fibers

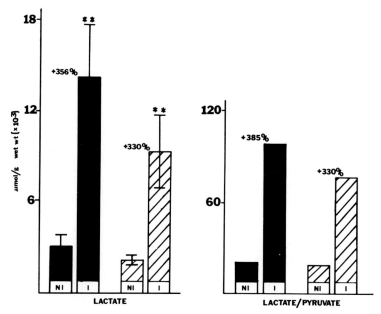

FIG. 2. The effect of diltiazem on tissue lactate levels and redox state. The drug lessens the increase in myocardial lactate concentration and the rise in lactate/pyruvate ratio. I, ischemic; NI, nonischemic; *, $0.05 < p < 0.10$; **, $p < 0.05$.

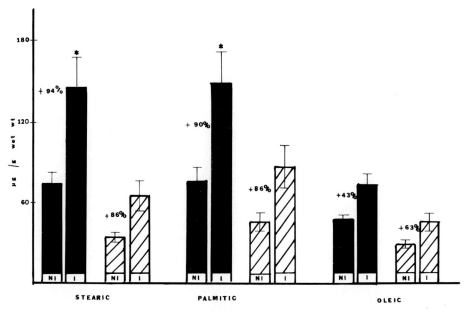

FIG. 3. The effect of diltiazem on myocardial free fatty acid (FFA). Although the difference in FFA between ischemic (I) and nonischemic (NI) remains on administration of the drug, diltiazem results in a diminution in FFA concentration in both I and NI tissues. *, $0.05 < p < 0.1$; **, $p < 0.05$.

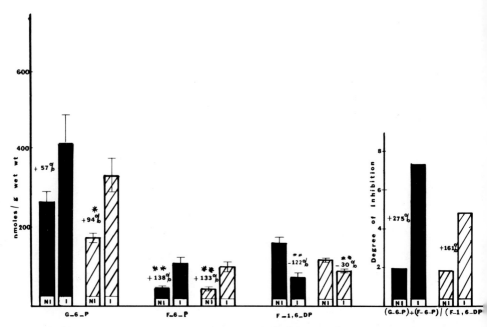

FIG. 4. The effect of diltiazem on glycolytic flux through phosphofructokinase. The drug relieves the inhibition of this enzyme and results in an increasing glycolytic flux. I, ischemic; NI, nonischemic; *, $0.05 < p < 0.1$; **, $p < 0.05$.

by 52 and 61% of nonischemic levels, respectively. In addition, t_o was prolonged by 90% in the ischemic fibers (Fig. 5). These changes were much less in fibers prepared from ischemic tissue in the diltiazem-treated dogs (Fig. 5). P_o was only 27% lower in ischemic fibers than in nonischemic, and dp/dt_{max} was reduced only 31%. In addition, values for t_o were only 22% higher in ischemic fibers than in nonischemic fibers in the animals treated with diltiazem.

In contrast to these marked effects, diltiazem did not lessen the effect of ischemia on mitochondrial respiration (Fig. 6). Mitochondrial oxygen consumption was reduced by roughly 15 to 30% of nonischemic levels in both groups. The greatest reduction was found with the substrate that directs electrons into site 1 of the electron transport chain (glutamate-oxalacetate). Mitochondrial respiratory control index was also reduced to a greater degree with this susbtrate. Diltiazem had no effect on mitochondrial calcium binding (Fig. 7).

These experiments, therefore, demonstrated that the administration of diltiazem lessened the effects of ischemia in several ways, including diminished breakdown of ATP in the ischemic region, improved glycolytic flux, increased contractility of isolated ischemic heart muscle fibers, and lower tissue levels of lactate and free fatty acids.

The reasons for these beneficial effects of this calcium antagonist have been alluded to above. Apparently, diltiazem, like other calcium antagonists, blocks

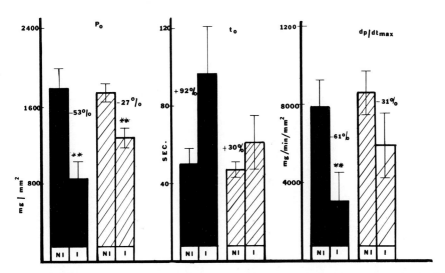

FIG. 5. Diltiazem increases contractility of glycerinated heart muscle fibers from ischemic (I) areas. **, $p < 0.05$.

contraction and produces a negative inotropic effect. Consequently, less ATP is consumed, and cardiac oxygen requirements diminish.

It has been recognized that resumption of coronary flow following regional myocardial ischemia often results in a paradoxical extension of the damage

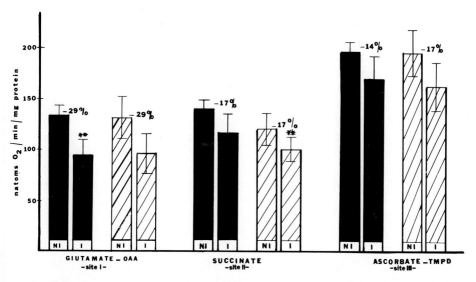

FIG. 6. Diltiazem has no effect on mitochondrial respiration after 60 min of ischemia. I, ischemic; NI, nonischemic; **, $p < 0.05$; control (no drug) and diltiazem (ischemia + diltiazem) as in other figures.

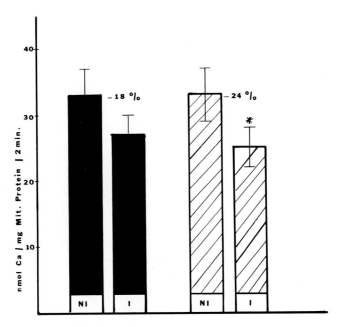

FIG. 7. Diltiazem has no effect on mitochondrial calcium binding after 60 min of ischemia. I, ischemic; NI, nonischemic; *, $0.05 < p < 0.1$.

produced by ischemia alone (16,21). This effect may be the result of a number of factors, many interrelated, including exhaustion of substrates, lowered pH, denaturation of enzymes, alterations in membrane permeability, and mitochondrial defects (18). Shen and Jennings (36) first proposed that reestablishment of flow following regional ischemia leads to cell swelling, development of contraction bands, and possible accumulation of calcium phosphate by the mitochondria. Hearse (16) has recently followed this up by proposing that the damage that accompanies the sudden readmission of molecular oxygen is the result of a massive energy-dependent influx of calcium ions into the mitochondrial matrix. This influx is thought to occur as an alternative to oxidative phosphorylation. This reoxygenation phenomenon may bear a close relationship to the calcium paradox described by Zimmerman (41), in which reinstitution of calcium ions to calcium-free perfusate results in diminished contractility and disappearance of electrical activity.

Mitochondrial dysfunction plays a predominant role in the production of this phenomenon. In examining the role of these organelles under these circumstances, Weishaar et al. (38) found that the severity of ischemia determines the degree of mitochondrial damage accompanying reperfusion. Reperfusion following moderate ischemia increased ATP and CP levels in the ischemic–reperfused region, as compared to levels of these metabolites following ischemia alone. Reperfusion following severe ischemia, however, led to a marked reduction

TABLE 2. *Effect of diltiazem administration on mitochondrial respiration (glutamate-oxalacetate) following regional myocardial ischemia (60 min) plus reperfusion (15 min)*

Group	ADP/O[a,b]	Q_{O_2}[a,c]—state 3	Q_{O_2}[a,c]—state 4
Control (no drug)			
Nonischemic ($n = 9$)	2.7 ± 0.1	152 ± 16	33 ± 5
Ischemic–reperfused ($n = 10$)	2.6 ± 0.1	82 ± 13	25 ± 6
± %	-4%	-46%[d]	-24%
Diltiazem			
Diltiazem given prior to reperfusion)			
Nonischemic ($n = 6$)	2.7 ± 0.1	132 ± 21	23 ± 4
Ischemic–reperfused ($n = 6$)	2.7 ± 0.1	108 ± 15	21 ± 3
± %	—	-22%	-10%

[a] Data represent the mean ± SE of the number of samples in parentheses.
[b] ADP/O = ratio of nanomoles of ADP phosphorylated per nanoatoms of oxygen consumed.
[c] Q_{O_2} = nmoles of oxygen consumed per minute per milligram of mitochondrial protein during active (state 3) and resting (state 4) respiration.
[d] $p < 0.05$.

in ATP in the ischemic–reperfused region. A similar trend was evident for mitochondrial oxygen consumption (Q_{O_2}) and mitochondrial calcium binding (38).

Experiments were therefore performed to study the effect of diltiazem on mitochondrial respiration and on mitochondrial calcium binding and uptake during ischemia and after 60 min of ischemia followed by reperfusion. Table 2 illustrates that the drug partially counteracted the effect of ischemia on mitochondrial Q_{O_2} (state 3). Reflow for 15 min after 60 min of ischemia reduced Q_{O_2} by 46%, while diltiazem resulted in some reversal of the defect. Table 3

TABLE 3. *Effect of diltiazem administration on mitochondrial Ca^{2+} binding following regional myocardial ischemia (60 min) and reperfusion (15 min)[a]*

	Time of binding		
Group	1 min	2 min	3 min
Control (no drug)			
Nonischemic ($n = 9$)	27 ± 6	42 ± 2	43 ± 3
Ischemic–reperfused ($n = 9$)	24 ± 3	27 ± 3	28 ± 2
± %	-11%	-36%	-35%
Diltiazem (diltiazem given prior to reperfusion)			
Nonischemic ($n = 4$)	21 ± 5	34 ± 6	44 ± 6
Ischemic–reperfused ($n = 4$)	20 ± 3	31 ± 5	40 ± 5
± %	-5%	-10%	-13%

[a] Data represent the mean ± SE of the number of samples in parentheses. Calcium binding expressed as nmoles Ca^{2+} bound/milligram of mitochondrial protein.

illustrates that mitochondrial calcium binding was markedly reduced by ischemia alone but that this deficit was reversed by diltiazem.

SUMMARY

The effect of antianginal drugs on systemic and myocardial blood flow and on myocardial metabolism was examined. In addition, emphasis was placed on the effect of a calcium antagonist, diltiazem, on myocardial ischemia and on the metabolic effects of reperfusion of the ischemic myocardium. The antianginal drugs were divided into three groups: (a) Those that act primarily on the redistribution of blood; (b) beta blockers; and (c) calcium antagonists. In group a, nitroglycerin and a new drug—molsidomin—affect primarily the capacity and compliance of the systemic venous system. Nitroglycerin also alters the endo-/epicardial perfusion ratio of the ischemic myocardium. No metabolic changes in heart muscle following the administration of these drugs could be demonstrated. In group b, beta blockers diminish myocardial contractility and heart rate via beta receptors. Propranolol also possesses a direct effect on myocardial substrate metabolism; it increases myocardial glucose and diminishes myocardial fatty acid extraction. In group c, calcium antagonists result in blockage of Ca^{2+} movement through the sarcolemma, thus producing a negative inotropic effect. All antianginal drugs, regardless of their specific effect, result in diminished myocardial oxygen demands and oxygen consumption. Diltiazem, a calcium antagonist, effectively counteracts some of the effects of acute myocardial ischemia. It lessened the fall in ATP and diminished tissue levels of lactate and increased glycolytic flux. In addition, as compared to the control, it improved myocardial contractility in glycerinated heart muscle fibers. Diltiazem also reduced some of the damaging effects of reperfusion following myocardial ischemia.

ACKNOWLEDGMENTS

This work was supported by grants from the Margaret W. and Herbert Hoover, Jr., Foundation and the Council for Tobacco Research–U.S.A., Inc.

REFERENCES

1. Ahlquist, R. P. (1948): Study of the adrenotropic receptors. *Am. J. Physiol.,* 153:586–600.
2. Becker, L. C., Fortuin, N. J., and Pitt, B. (1971): Effect of ischemia and antianginal drugs on the distribution of radioactive microspheres in the canine left ventricle. *Circ. Res.,* 21:263–269.
3. Bing, R. J., Bender, S. R., Dunn, M. I., Fry, G. A., Fuller, W. M., Liu, S. C. K., Miller, H. S., Moses, J. W., Ritzman, L. W., Segal, J. P., Shugoll, G. I., Tillmanns, H., and Wallace, A. (1974): Antianginal effects of chromonar. *Clin. Pharmacol. Ther.,* 16:4–13.
4. Bing, R. J., and Hellberg, K. (1972): Coronary blood flow in relation to angina pectoris. *Circulation,* 46:1146–1154.
5. Black, J. W., Crowther, A. F., Shanks, R. G., Smith, L. H., and Dornhorst, A. C. (1964): A new adrenergic beta-receptor antagonist. *Lancet,* 1:1080–1081.
6. Brunton, T. L. (1867): On the use of nitrite of amyl in angina pectoris. *Lancet,* 2:97.

7. Cohen, A., Gallagher, J. P., Luebs, E. D., Varga, Z., Yamanaka, J., Zaleski, E. J., Bluemchen, G., and Bing, R. J. (1965): The quantitative determination of coronary flow with a positron emitter (Rubidium-84). *Circulation,* 32:636–649.
8. Cohen, M. V., Sonnenblick, E. H., and Kirk, E. S. (1976): Comparative effects of nitroglycerin and isosorbide dinitrate on coronary collateral vessels and ischemic myocardium in dogs. *Am. J. Cardiol.,* 37:244–249.
9. Crevey, B. J., Langer, G. A., and Frank, J. S. (1978): Role of Ca^{2+} in maintenance of rabbit myocardial cell membrane structural and functional integrity. *J. Mol. Cell. Cardiol.,* 10:1081–1100.
10. Essex, H. E., Wegria, R. G. E., Herrick, J. F., and Mann, F. C. (1940): The effect of certain drugs on the coronary blood flow of the trained dog. *Am. Heart J.,* 19:554–565.
11. Ferrer, M. I., Bradley, S. E., Wheeler, H. O., Enson, Y., Preisig, R., Brickner, P. W., Conroy, R. J., and Harvey, R. M. (1966): Some effects of nitroglycerin upon the splanchnic, pulmonary, and systemic circulations. *Circulation,* 33:357–373.
12. Fleckenstein, A. (1971): Specific inhibitors and promoters of calcium action in the excitation–contraction coupling of heart muscle and their role in the prevention or production of myocardial lesions. In: *Calcium and the Heart,* edited by P. Harris and L. H. Opie, pp. 135–188. Academic Press, New York.
13. Gillam, P. M. S., and Prichard, B. N. C. (1965): Use of propranolol in angina pectoris. *Br. Med. J.,* 2:337–339.
14. Gross, J. G., and Winbury, M. M. (1973): Beta-adrenergic blockade on intramyocardial distribution of coronary blood flow. *J. Pharmacol. Exp. Ther.,* 187:451–464.
15. Harigaya, S., and Schwartz, A. (1969): Rate of calcium binding and uptake in normal animal and failing human cardiac muscle. Membrane vesicles (relaxing system) and mitochondria. *Circ. Res.,* 25:781–794.
16. Hearse, D. J. (1977): Reperfusion of the ischemic myocardium. *J. Mol. Cell. Cardiol.,* 9:605–616 (Editorial).
17. Horwitz, L. D., Gorlin, R., Taylor, W. J., and Kemp, H. G. (1971): Effects of nitroglycerin on regional myocardial blood flow in coronary artery disease. *J. Clin. Invest.,* 50:1578–1584.
18. Jennings, R. B. (1976): Relationship of acute ischemia to functional defects and irreversibility. Discussion. *Circulation (Suppl. I),* 53:26–29.
19. Kane, J. J., Murphy, M. L., Bissett, J. K., de Soyza, N., Doherty, J. T., and Straub, K. D. (1975): Mitochondrial function, oxygen extraction, epicardial S–T segment changes and tritiated digoxin distribution after reperfusion of ischemic myocardium. *Am. J. Cardiol.,* 36:218–224.
20. Katz, A. M. (1977): *Physiology of the Heart.* Raven Press, New York.
21. Kloner, R. A., Ganote, C. E., and Jennings, R. B. (1974): The "no-reflow" phenomenon after temporary coronary occlusion in the dog. *J. Clin. Invest.,* 54:1496–1508.
22. Kloner, R. A., Reimer, K. A., and Jennings, R. B. (1976): Distribution of coronary collateral flow in acute myocardial ischaemic injury: Effect of propranolol. *Cardiovasc. Res.,* 10:81–90.
23. Marchetti, G., Merlo, L., and Noseda, V. (1968): Myocardial uptake of free fatty acids and carbohydrates after beta-adrenergic blockade. *Am. J. Cardiol.,* 22:370–374.
24. Mueller-Buchholtz, E. R., Loesch, H. M., Grund, E., and Lochner, W. (1977): Effect of alpha-adrenergic receptor stimulation on integrated systemic venous bed. *Pfluegers Arch.,* 370:247–252.
25. Mueller, H. S., Ayres, S. M., Religa, A., and Evans, R. G. (1974): Propranolol in the treatment of acute myocardial infarction: Effect on myocardial oxygenation and hemodynamics. *Circulation,* 49:1078–1087.
26. Mueller, O., and Rørvik, K. (1958): Haemodynamic consequences of coronary heart disease with observations during anginal pain and on the effect of nitroglycerine. *Br. Heart J.,* 20:302–310.
27. Nayler, W. G., McInnes, I., Swann, J. B., Carson, V., and Lowe, T. E. (1967): Effects of propranolol, a beta-adrenergic antagonist, on blood flow in the coronary and other vascular fields. *Am. Heart J.,* 73:207–216.
28. Neely, J. R., Whitmer, J. T., and Rovetto, M. J. (1975): Effect of coronary blood flow on glycolytic flux and intracellular pH in isolated rat hearts. *Circ. Res.,* 37:733–751.
29. Ogawa, K., Gudbjarnason, S., and Bing, R. J. (1967): Nitroglycerin (glyceryl trinitrate) as a monoamine oxidase inhibitor. *J. Pharmacol. Exp. Ther.,* 155:449–455.
30. Opie, L. H., and Thomas, M. (1976): Propranolol and experimental myocardial infarctions: Substrate effects. *Postgraduate Med. J. (Suppl. 4),* 52:124–132.

31. Robin, E., Cowan, C., Puri, P., Ganguly, S., DeBoyrie, E., Martinez, M., Stock, T., and Bing, R. J. (1967): A comparative study of nitroglycerin and propranolol. *Circulation,* 36:175–186.
32. Ross, J., Frahm, C. J., and Braunwald, E. (1961): Influence of carotid baroreceptors and vasoactive drugs on systemic vascular volume and venous distensibility. *Circ. Res.,* 9:75–82.
33. Sarma, J. S. M., Ikeda, S., Fischer, R., Maruyama, Y., Weishaar, R., and Bing, R. J. (1976): Biochemical and contractile properties of heart muscle after prolonged alcohol administration. *J. Mol. Cell. Cardiol.* 8:951–972.
34. Schartl, M., Botsch, H., and Rutsch, W. (1978): Einfluss von Molsidomin auf Parameter des Niederdrucksystems. Haemodynamische, Venenverschlussplethysmographische und Szintigraphische Untersuchungen. Presented at the meeting on *New Aspects in Therapy of Ischemic Heart Disease.* Munich.
35. Schwartz, A., Wood, J. M., Allen, J. C., Bornet, E. P., Entman, M. L., Goldstein, M. A., Sordahl, L. A., and Suzuki, M. (1973): Biochemical and morphologic correlates of cardiac ischemia. I. Membrane systems. *Am. J. Cardiol.,* 32:46–61.
36. Shen, A. C., and Jennings, R. B. (1972): Kinetics of calcium accumulation in acute myocardial ischemic injury. *Am. J. Pathol.,* 67:441–452.
37. Srivastava, S. C., Dewar, H. A., and Newell, D. J. (1964): Double-blind trial of propranolol (Inderal) in angina of effort. *Br. Med. J.,* 2:724–725.
38. Weishaar, R., and Bing, R. J. (1979): The effect of diltiazem, a calcium-antagonist, on myocardial ischemia. *Am. J. Cardiol. (in press).*
39. Weishaar, R., Sarma, J. S. M., Maruyama, Y., Fischer, R., and Bing, R. J. (1977): Regional blood flow, contractility and metabolism in early myocardial infarction. *Cardiology,* 62:2–20.
40. Williams, J. F., Glick, G., and Braunwald, E. (1965): Studies on cardiac dimensions in intact unanesthetized man. V. Effects of nitroglycerin. *Circulation,* 32:767–771.
41. Zimmermann, A. N. E., Daems, W., Huelsmann, W. C., Snyder, J., Wisse, E. and Durrer, D. (1967): Morphological changes of heart muscle caused by successive perfusion with calcium-free and calcium-containing solutions (calcium paradox). *Cardiovasc. Res.,* 1:201–209.

Ischemic Myocardium and Antianginal Drugs,
edited by M. M. Winbury and Y. Abiko.
Raven Press, New York © 1979.

Effect of Medical and Surgical Therapy on Regional Myocardial Ischemia

W. Bleifeld, W. Kupper, D. Mathey, and P. Hanrath

*Department of Cardiology, Medical Clinic II, University Hospital Eppendorf,
D-2000 Hamburg, West Germany*

Pathological studies (72) and the evaluation of infarct size in man (5,8,88) have demonstrated that the size of an acute infarct determines the pump function in terms of cardiac output and filling pressure, the frequency and severity of cardiac arrhythmias (80), and, accordingly, the prognosis (88). Thus, besides the maintenance of electrical stability and sufficient pump function, the final goal in the therapy of acute myocardial infarction is to minimize infarct size (16). In looking at this goal, first, methods for the evaluation of ischemia will be critically reviewed and second, the results of different pharmaceutical and surgical interventions in the clinical setting will be discussed.

METHODS FOR THE EVALUATION OF ISCHEMIA

Of the numerous techniques to evaluate extent and degree of myocardial ischemia used in animal experiments, only a limited number have been introduced into clinical use (Table 1): (a) biochemical markers; (b) precordial electrocardiogram (EKG) mapping; and (c) myocardial imaging. In addition, alterations of local contraction obtained quantitatively from angiograms in the control state and after pharmaceutical or electrical interventions (28,39,48,51) have been used.

Biochemical Markers

Creatine Kinase and Creatine Kinase–MB Isoenzyme

It is now widely accepted that serial creatine kinase (CK) measurements allow the best *in vivo* estimate of infarct size (6,68,88). This has been shown by a good correlation between calculated infarct size and that measured at autopsy (8). Moreover, a similarly good correlation was observed when the area of the akinetic region in the postinfarction left ventricular angiogram was related to the infarct size calculated from serial CK measurement (82,92). Although the use of the CK–MB isoenzyme which originates almost exclusively from the heart muscle is preferable to the total CK, investigations from our own

TABLE 1. *Methods for assessment of myocardial ischemia*

---

1. Biochemical markers
   (a) CK:CK-MB
   (b) Lactate
   (c) Inosine, hypoxanthine
   (d) In combination with coronary sinus flow
2. Precordial EKG mapping
3. Myocardial imaging
4. Evaluation of ventricular angiogram

---

laboratory have shown an excellent correlation between infarct size calculated from the cumulative activity of the MB fraction and that of the total CK. Only in rare cases of noncoronary obstructive myocardial necrosis may a rise of the serum CK–MB concentration be observed. This reflects the fact that the sensitivity of CK–MB elevation for the diagnosis of myocardial infarction is nearly 100% (44) but the specificity is considerably lower. In clinical practice, however, total CK can be used for the estimation of infarct size if extracardiac sources (e.g., in cardiac standstill) or noncoronary myocardial necroses are eliminated.

Three points useful in the diagnosis and evaluation of the course of the disease can be obtained from serial CK determinations. First, the cumulative activity can be expressed as gram equivalents of destroyed myocardium, indicating the size of the infarct. Second, an extension of the infarct can be diagnosed by another rise of the CK or a late maximum (60% of all cases) (60). Third, infarct size may be predicted by extrapolation from the values in the initial 2 to 7 hr (86), thus enabling the comparison of actual and predicted infarct size and, by this, the evaluation of the effect of therapeutic intervention.

Lactate

Although the pathways of metabolic derangement in an ischemic myocardial cell and, accordingly, the indicators of ischemia, are well known (32,42,69), this knowledge could not be transferred to the clinical setting for the following reasons. First, some of the metabolic products that develop during ischemia in a cell may pass into the blood only if there is a defect in the cell membrane. Thus, although the myocardium is definitely ischemic, the ischemia cannot be detected from alteration of the venous, arterial, or even the coronary sinus blood. Second, the detection of other metabolic products (i.e., adenosine diphosphate or adenosine) that pass into the blood requires difficult biochemical methods that are not, at present, available in hospitals. Nevertheless, although the occurrence of pathological concentrations of lactate may be caused by factors other than ischemia (70) and although exercise stress testing makes the use of lactate assays impossible, the determination of lactate is the simplest and most often used method for the evaluation of ischemic states (spontaneous, in myocardial infarction, or induced by electrical stimulation), and lactate production correlates well with the development of angina, ST segment alterations, and local contraction abnormalities (73).

Inosine and Hypoxanthine

Other biochemical markers that have also been used recently in the clinical setting are inosine and hypoxanthine (37). Whereas in pigs the sensitivity of inosine and hypoxanthine is higher than that of lactate (37), in dogs and in humans it has not been shown to be preferable to lactate. The advantage of using inosine during exercise stress testing may be outweighed by the difficult biochemical procedure necessary for its determination (43).

Biochemical Markers in Conjunction with Coronary Sinus Blood Flow Measurement

Marked progress in this field has been made by the combination of coronary sinus blood flow measurement using the Ganz thermodilution technique and the determination of the biochemical markers mentioned above (31). By using a double-thermistor catheter positioned with the tip at the inflow of the left anterior descending vein into the great cardiac vein (Fig. 1), blood flow and

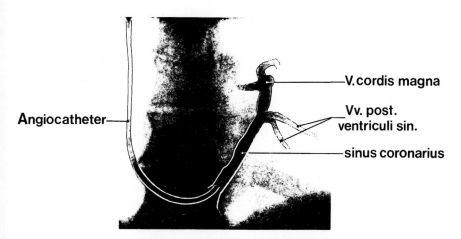

FIG. 1. Coronary venous angiogram illustrating technique for combined coronary sinus blood measurement and blood sampling. A thermistor catheter is introduced into the coronary sinus positioned with the tip at the inflow of left anterior descending vein and a second thermistor at the mouth of the coronary sinus. A venous angiogram serves to investigate the local anatomical conditions.

lactate level from the anterior wall of the left ventricle can be determined in addition to the total coronary sinus blood flow and lactate level changes.

Precordial EKG Mapping

The second method—precordial EKG mapping (46)—has been derived from animal experiments (7,9,55,76) and is based on the fact that the log of serum CK is inversely related to height of the ST segment elevation and to the sum of the change in the R wave (ΔR) and the change of the Q wave (ΔQ) 24 hr after myocardial infarction (46). As has long been known by experienced clinicians, however, there are certainly some limitations. A principal disadvantage of the method is that only infarctions of the anterior and lateral wall can be evaluated. The distance between the epicardial lead recordings and EKG maps obtained from the chest wall may further reduce the sensitivity and, accordingly, the specificity. Factors other than ischemia may influence the ST segment: Alterations in ion concentrations (particularly potassium), temperature changes, drugs such as quinidine and digitalis, and epicardial injury due to pericarditis are well known to affect the ST segment and must be taken into account. Arrhythmias, increased heart rate, and sympathetic stimulation of the heart may produce further changes (12,33,41,46). Moreover, even in an individual patient, ST segment elevation cannot be taken in every case as an expression of myocardial necrosis; only in the presence of a CK increase does it indicate myocardial

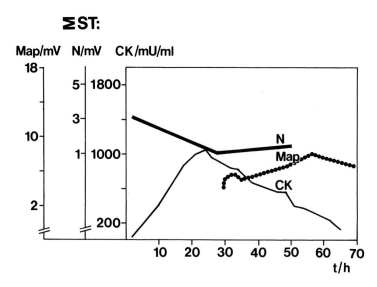

FIG. 2. Mean sum of ST segment elevation from the precordial mapping [MAP *(dots)*], the conventional 12-lead EKG [N *(thick line)*], and the CK concentration *(thin line)* in a case of atrial fibrillation with tachycardia 35 hr after infarction. While CK declines normally, there is a rise of the ST segment in the MAP, indicating ischemia without necrosis.

necrosis (Fig. 2). As an example, the ST segment may elevate during an episode of tachycardia without an elevation of the CK or CK–MB activity. With these limitations and pitfalls in mind, a rough and, therefore, only qualitative evaluation of the effect of an intervention is possible by the use of precordial EKG mapping (46).

Devices were constructed with 36 to 48 fixed precordial leads positioned on the body surface so that the first line runs along the right sternal border beginning in the second intercostal space. In our laboratory, a computer is attached via an x–y digitizer that evaluates the parameters indicated in Fig. 3 and feeds them into the computer. In this way, the complete examination of a 36 precordial EKG takes about 10 min.

Using precordial mapping as an indicator of ischemia, one must know the natural course of the ST segment changes in the acute phase of a myocardial infarction. In our experience, the rise of the ST segment begins after 3 to 5 min and reaches its maximum at about 5 to 6 hr after the onset of symptoms (66,85).

Q waves develop in the second hour after the onset of clinical signs and are completed within 12 hr (84). Myocardial extension occurs in about 60% of patients with acute myocardial infarction, as evaluated from precordial mapping (77). Recent studies (33) have shown that CK–MB activity, which may serve as a reference method because of the characteristic type of time course, does not correlate, in uncomplicated infarction, with the time course of the sum of ST segment elevation and that several discrepancies can occur in complicated infarction. In addition, the maximum ST segment elevation is fully developed before the maximal increase of CK–MB.

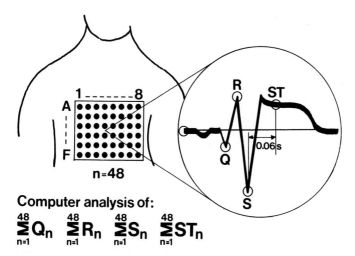

FIG. 3. Schematic drawing of the 48-lead precordial EKG mapping. The parameters summarized at the bottom are evaluated from the EKG *(right)*.

Myocardial Imaging Through the Use of Radionuclides

In the past few years, radionuclides (18,71,78,79) have been introduced into clinical use to detect, localize, and quantitate an ischemic area. Biphasic (rest and exercise stress test) [201]thallium scintigraphy enables differentiation between reversible and irreversible ischemic areas. A reversible defect is defined as occurring only during stress and angina, whereas an irreversible ischemic area occurs also at rest (62). Although recent pathological studies (89) have demonstrated that normal myocardium is also found in an irreversible [201]thallium defect, the clinical relevance of differentiating between the two types of defect is that the chances of improving and/or normalizing the coronary blood flow and contractile function by coronary artery bypass surgery are greater in the case of a reversible defect than an irreversible defect.

In this context, the correlation of [201]thallium scintigraphy to ST segment changes, as an indicator of ischemia, and to local contraction abnormalities is of interest. A pathological [201]thallium scintigram was found in 26 of 32 dyskinetic areas, in 13 of 20 akinetic areas, and in only 20% (27 of 138) of the normal contracting areas (reversible, 14.5%; irreversible, 5.5%) (Table 2). When comparing the thallium scintigram with the results of the exercise stress test EKG (Table 3) in patients with coronary heart disease proved by coronary angiogram, of the 30 patients who were positive in the EKG, all had a thallium defect after exercise. From the 27 patients negative in the EKG, 19 (67%) had thallium defects after stress, and of the other eight patients negative in the thallium scintigram, only two had significant ($> 75\%$ of the diameter) stenosis. Thus (a) the [201]thallium scintigram has greater sensitivity than the exercise stress test EKG; and (b) it provides an additional tool to verify not only ischemia, but also the localization and extent of ischemia.

Evaluation of Ventricular Angiogram

Since the observation of Tennant and Wiggers (90) that minutes after ligation of a coronary artery there is a substantial loss of contraction, the dependence

TABLE 2. *Comparisons of [201]thallium scintigrams to regional wall motion in left ventricular angiogram*

Regions in the LV[a] angiogram	Results in the [201]Th scintigram[b]		
	Ir. defect	R. defect	Normal
Normal	7	20	111
Hypokinetic	18	20	20
Akinetic	9	4	7
Dyskinetic	20	6	6

[a] LV, left ventricular.
[b] Ir. defect, irreversible defect; R. defect, reversible defect.

TABLE 3. *Comparison of biphasic [201]thalium scintigraphy with exercise stress test EKG*

Exercise test EKG	[201]Thalium defect		Coronary stenoses
	After exercise	At rest	
30 (+)	30 (+)	{ 27 (−) { 3 (+)	{ 27 (+) { 3 (+)
27 (−)	{ 19 (+) { { 8 (−)	{ 9 (+) { 10 (−) { 2 (+) { 6 (−)	{ 9 (+) { 10 (+) { 2 (+) { 6 (−)
5 LBB[a]	5 (+)	{ 3 (+) { 2 (−)	{ 3 (+) { 2 (+)

[a] LBB, left bundle branch block.

of the contractile behavior on the supply of oxygen has been overlooked. Recent studies (58), however, have demonstrated that the loss of mechanical function following biochemical derangement (loss of ATP and creatine phosphokinase) is the earliest and most sensitive indicator of ischemia. When coronary blood flow was decreased 75%, the mechanical action was markedly impaired. Following these results, clinicians used the shortening of the lateral axis calculated from the angiogram to evaluate the degree of mechanical impairment at rest, after nitroglycerin (17) or postextrasystolic potentiation (28,39). Areas contracting after the application of nitroglycerin or of a postextrasystolic beat were regarded as ischemic but viable and, therefore, as having the potential for improved or normal contraction after coronary bypass surgery. Thus the evaluation of angiograms is widely used for the detection of ischemic areas.

RESULTS OF PHARMACEUTICAL INTERVENTION ON THE EXTENT AND DEGREE OF ISCHEMIA

Pharmaceutical Interventions

Using serial CK determinations and cumulative CK activity, Roberts et al. (80) reduced infarct size by 25% in a subgroup of infarctions with hypertension when the elevated blood pressure was decreased by trimetaphan. In contrast, Varonkov et al. (91) found that strophantin caused extension of an acute infarction. Both studies were performed on the basis of a prediction of the infarct mass from the CK values for the first 6 to 7 hr. Recently, the observation of Miura et al. (67) that propanolol reduces the infarct size in closed-chest anesthetized dogs has also been noted in man (75). In a randomized trial in 95 patients, 27% of those treated orally with 320 mg propanolol (over 27 hr) after a loading dose of 0.1 mg/kg i.v. had lower peak-measured enzyme levels than 19 untreated patients. Although these patients entered the study within 4 hr after the onset of clinical signs, no significant difference was found when treatment was initiated after 4 hr.

These results are of utmost importance since they show that therapy must be initiated as early as possible and, on the basis of serum enzyme measurements, is ineffective after 4 to 6 hr. This latter fact may reflect that this method may be insensitive for detecting only small alterations of infarct size, which can be evaluated by other methods, such as precordial mapping or coronary sinus lactate sampling. However, the question is still open.

The effect of nitroglycerin on total coronary blood flow and the central and peripheral hemodynamics in coronary artery disease is well known. In our own laboratory, we investigated the effect of nitroglycerin on total and regional (outflow from the left anterior descending vein) myocardial blood flow (see Fig. 1) and metabolism at rest and during pacing-induced angina in patients with severe stenosis ($> 80\%$) of the left anterior descending artery. While total coronary blood flow and great cardiac vein blood flow were unchanged, lactate production changed to extraction as a consequence of a significant decrease in the pressure–rate product ratio (Fig. 4). These results show that (a) nitroglycerin does not increase coronary artery blood flow in severe coronary artery stenosis; and (b) the beneficial effects of nitroglycerin on the degree of angina are produced by the reduction of the pressure–rate product and the decrease of left ventricular filling pressure in the presence of an unchanged or even slightly diminished great cardiac vein and total coronary sinus blood flow.

Only in the subgroup of Prinzmetal angina may nitroglycerin exert a direct effect on the epicardial arteries by abolishing a spasm (57). However, in the

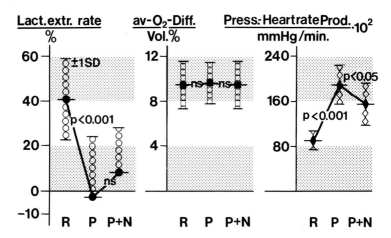

FIG. 4. Effect of atrial stimulation (P) and pretreatment with nitroglycerin (N) in the presence of pacing (P + N) on lactate extraction rate, atrioventricular oxygen difference, and pressure–rate product compared to the control state (R). SD, standard deviation. NS, not significant.

long-term prevention of recurrent spasms, calcium antagonists seem to be preferable (35).

Nitroglycerin has also been shown to improve regional myocardial function
(17,23,34), but only in those regions in which the loss, on histopathological
examination, was less than 10%. Those regions not reacting with an increased
contraction exhibited significant fibrosis (11).

With the same technique, the effect of pindolol—a selective β_1-receptor blocking agent—was studied in patients with coronary heart disease at rest and during
atrial stimulation. After pretreatment with 6 μg pindolol/kg, no significant effects
could be observed in the total group of 18 patients. When the total group
was divided into two subgroups, one with and one without pathological lactate
extraction during stimulation, different results were obtained. In those patients
without lactate production during stimulation, pressure–rate product and, accordingly, myocardial oxygen consumption were favorably affected and coronary
blood flow decreased, with lactate extraction unchanged (Fig. 5). In the subgroup
of lactate-producing patients (Fig. 6), however, there was a marked but not
significant reduction of the negative lactate extraction from −31 to −12%. In
addition, five of the eight patients exhibited no angina at the same stimulation
rate.

Similar results have recently been obtained by Jackson et al. (35) in that
tolamolol (0.15 mg/kg) or propanolol (0.1 mg/kg) resulted in a significant increase of lactate and glucose extraction; an increase in tolerance time and a

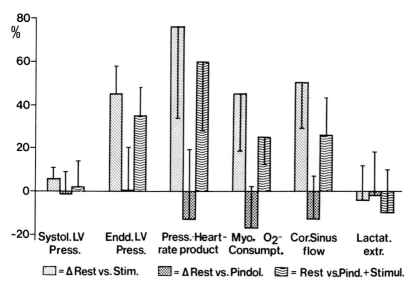

FIG. 5. Effect of pindolol on various parameters of left ventricular hemodynamics in a subgroup
of patients ($n = 10$) with coronary heart disease who produced no lactate during atrial stimulation. EF = 68 ± 6%.

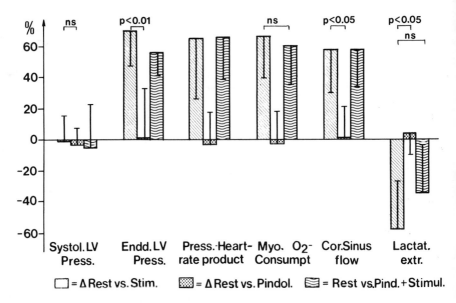

FIG. 6. Effect of pindolol on various parameters of left ventricular hemodynamics in a subgroup of patients ($n = 8$) with lactate production during atrial stimulation. (For details, see text.) EF $= 47 \pm 23\%$.

decrease of the ST segment depression was observed in the presence of unaltered left ventricular hemodynamics (81). From these results, it can be concluded that β-blocking agents may change angina threshold and lactate metabolism without affecting the coronary sinus blood flow or myocardial oxygen consumption. This has also been advocated by Armstrong et al. (2).

Most investigations of the effect of drugs on the extent of ischemia have been performed using epicardial (72,78) or precordial EKG mapping (46). In an experiment conducted by Come et al. (25), orally administered isosorbide dinitrate exhibited a significant reduction in the number of affected leads and in the mean sum of ST segment elevation. Similar results have been obtained for nitroglycerin in a study by Maroko et al. (55). In a study by Bussmann et al. (19), however, nitroglycerin had no effect on the cumulative CK activity in the presence of marked hemodynamic improvement, which could be explained by the low sensitivity of CK as a marker of ischemia. Obviously, the effect of nitroglycerin on arterial pressure and heart rate may result in adverse effects, as shown in a study by Borer et al. (13). When these investigators stabilized blood pressure during nitroglycerin, the ST segment elevation was further reduced. Therefore, blood pressure and heart rate must be watched carefully.

In another study nitroglycerin and sodium nitroprusside were compared. Both drugs exerted similar hemodynamic results, but the ST segment elevation was favorably influenced only by nitroglycerin (54). This result might be explained by the fact that in radioactive microsphere studies, blood flow was redistributed from the nonischemic to the ischemic areas by nitroglycerin but not by sodium nitroprusside (3). However, other studies have demonstrated a favorable effect of nitroprusside on regional flow (52) in addition to the good results obtained in treating severe left heart failure (47).

Surgical Interventions—Coronary Artery Bypass Surgery

Ever since the introduction of coronary bypass surgery (CABS) (2,10,29, 49,63), the effect of the therapy has been evaluated by the relief from angina. There is no doubt that about 80% of the operated patients exhibit a marked improvement in their quality of life as evidenced by relief from angina and an increased working capacity (20,27). Except for cases of coronary artery disease with left main coronary artery stenosis, the effects on mortality and the functional state of the myocardium are still under debate (15). There is no doubt that, even in the presence of a totally occluded bypass, the patient may have become free of pain (24,53). Thus, relief from pain is no indicator of the improvement in coronary blood supply, which is the objective of the surgical procedure. All studies concerning the acute (6,8) and long-term course of an acute myocardial infarction (4) suggest that an increase in blood supply by CABS to the myocardium of a severely stenotic area improves the functional state and, accordingly, the pump function and reduces or alleviates cardiac arrhythmias, thereby leading to a reduction of mortality. Thus, it is of utmost importance to measure the effect of bypass surgery not only by the change in angina but also by the alteration in myocardial blood flow, myocardial metabolism, and functional state.

Therefore, we investigated the alteration of coronary sinus blood flow and lactate concentration in 12 patients before and 4 to 6 weeks after surgery. The mean results of eight of the patients are shown in Table 4. Coronary sinus blood flow at rest increased about 20% and flow during atrial stimulation increased about 90%, although a wide scattering was observed. Thus coronary reserve was elevated markedly.

Myocardial lactate extraction changed from a marked production of $-29 \pm 42\%$

TABLE 4. *Effect of coronary bypass surgery on coronary sinus blood flow and lactate*

	CSBF[a] (ml/min) (n = 8)		LE[b] (%) (n = 8)	
	Preop	Postop	Preop	Postop
Rest	94 ± 20	113 ± 22	26 ± 17	39 ± 14
Atrial stimulation	116 ± 34	225 ± 96	-29 ± 42 (n = 7)	8 ± 24

[a]CSBF, coronary sinus blood flow.
[b]LE, lactate extraction rate.

to an extraction of +8 ± 24%. Angina threshold increased from a heart rate of 123 to 148 beats/min. However, as seen from the large standard deviation, the results were not uniform. Whereas in some patients coronary reserve was enlarged, in others no increase was observed (Fig. 7). For example, patient 3 showed no increase in coronary blood flow at rest and during stimulation but showed no angina after increasing heart rate.

Similar results have been observed by Chatterjee et al. (21,22) in 18 patients studied before and after CABS. Coronary sinus blood flow increased from 111 ml/min at rest and 202 ml/min during stimulation before surgery to 152 and 266 ml/min, respectively, postoperatively. In seven patients with lactate production, six improved markedly. In three patients in whom lactate metabolism at the outflow of the anterior wall was investigated, this region showed a normalization both at rest and during maximal stimulation rate.

An increase in myocardial blood flow was also observed in the majority of patients with coronary artery bypass, when investigated by radioactive [133]xenon (24). There was no correlation between exercise tolerance and blood flow changes.

Although several reports have dealt with the improvement of pump function in terms of cardiac output, stroke volume, or stroke work, only recently has regional mechanical function been investigated. In a group of patients with single vessel disease with normal ventricular volumes and ejection fraction before and after bypass surgery, preoperative abnormalities in the wall motion were restored to normal (64).

A study by Levine et al. (50) correlated bypass patency and regional ventricular wall motion. There were directional changes in the increase of local and total arterial blood supply and changes in segmental wall motion and ejection fraction in either open or closed grafts corresponding with additional progression of

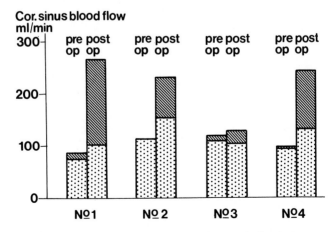

FIG. 7. Coronary reserve (CR) in 4 of 12 patients before and after bypass surgery during atrial stimulation *(lines)* and at rest *(dots)*. Although most of them exhibited a marked increase in CR, there was no improvement in patient 3.

the atherosclerotic disease. It was of interest that, despite a deterioration of mechanical function and graft closure, anginal symptoms decreased in nearly all patients, which is in agreement with Bloch et al. (10).

The improvement of regional mechanical function need not necessarily be obvious at rest (83). As Kent et al. (38) pointed out, the ejection fraction and exercise-induced wall motion abnormalities improved in most patients who also showed a symptomatic improvement.

From the presently available information regarding the effect of medical and surgical therapy on regional myocardial ischemia, one can conclude the following:

(a) At present, some methods are available in the clinical setting that are more or less sensitive and that should all be used, if possible, in the same patient group because they permit different views of the myocardium.

(b) There is no doubt that, in human studies, we require more parameters reflecting the myocardial metabolism to indicate when a cell or an area of the myocardium becomes ischemic or dies.

(c) Nitroglycerin, isosorbide dinitrate, and β-blocking agents reduce the degree of ischemia, but there is still a lack of information as to what extent (i.e., in grams of myocardial mass) they reduce ischemia. Moreover, the use of these drugs in humans requires the careful monitoring of other hemodynamic parameters, such as arterial pressure.

(d) Coronary bypass surgery can definitely increase coronary blood flow and reduce lactate production in addition to relieving angina. However, one should be aware that the latter is not necessarily a sign of improvement of the myocardial function. Furthermore, one should also realize that comprehensive studies are necessary to define in advance the candidate for bypass surgery.

ACKNOWLEDGMENTS

The authors thank Mrs. H. Zolldahn, Mrs. C. Freyer, Mrs. K. Maass, Mr. C. Hamm, and the staff of the catheterization laboratory for their assistance and Mrs. Minssen for her careful secretarial work.

REFERENCES

1. Apstein, C. S., Deckelbaum, L., Mueller, M., Hagopian, L., and Hood, W. B., Jr. (1977): Graded global ischemia and reperfusion. Cardiac function and lactate metabolism. *Circulation,* 55:864–872.
2. Armstrong, P. W., Chiong, M. A., and Parker, J. O. (1977): Effects of propanolol on the hemodynamic, coronary sinus blood flow and myocardial metabolic response to atrial pacing. *Am. J. Cardiol.,* 40:83–89.
3. Becker, L. C., Fortuin, N. J., and Pitt, B. (1971): Effect of ischemia and antianginal drugs on the distribution of radioactive microspheres in the canine left ventricle. *Circ. Res.,* 28:263–269.
4. Bleifeld, W., Hanrath, P., and Mathey, D. (1974): Akuter Myokardinfarkt. X. Veränderungen der Haemodynamik des rechten und linken Ventrikels vom akuten Stadium zur Rekonvaleszenz. *Dtsch. Med. Wochenschr.,* 99:1049–1057.

5. Bleifeld, W., Hanrath, P., and Mathey, D. (1976): Serial CPK determinations for evaluation of size and development of acute myocardial infarction. *Circulation (Suppl. I),* 53:I-108–I-111.
6. Bleifeld, W., Hanrath, P., Mathey, D., and Merx, W. (1974): Acute myocardial infarction. V. Left and right ventricular haemodynamics in cardiogenic shock. *Br. Heart J.,* 36:822–834.
7. Bleifeld, W., and Irnich, W. (1973): Methode zur epikardialen Ekg-Registrierung. *Z. Kardiol.,* 62:424–432.
8. Bleifeld, W., Mathey, D., Hanrath, P., Buss, H., and Effert, S. (1977): Infarct size estimated from serial creatine phosphokinase in relation to left ventricular hemodynamics. *Circulation,* 55:303–311.
9. Bleifeld, W., Wende, W., Bussmann, W. D., and Meyer, J. (1973): Influence of nitroglycerin on the size of experimental myocardial infarction. *Naunyn Schmiedebergs Arch. Pharmacol.,* 277:387–400.
10. Block, T. A., Murray, J. A., and English, M. T. (1977): Improvement in exercise performance after unsuccessful myocardial revascularization. *Am. J. Cardiol.,* 40:673–680.
11. Bodenheimer, M. M., Banka, V. S., Hermann, G. A., Trout, R. G., Pasdar, H., and Helfant, R. H. (1976): Reversible asynergy. Histopathologic and electrographic correlations in patients with coronary artery disease. *Circulation,* 53:792–796.
12. Boineau, J. P. (1971): Modification of infarct size. *Circulation,* 43:317 (letter).
13. Borer, J. S., Redwood, D. R., Levitt, B., Cagin, N., Bianchi, C., Vattin, H., and Epstein, St. E. (1975): Reduction in myocardial ischemia with nitroglycerin or nitroglycerin plus phenylephrine administered during acute myocardial infarction. *N. Engl. J. Med.,* 293:1008–1012.
14. Bourassa, M. G., Campeau, L., Bois, M. A., and Rico, O. (1969): Myocardial lactate metabolism at rest and during exercise in ischemic heart disease. *Am. J. Cardiol.,* 23:771–777.
15. Braunwald, E. (1978): Evaluation of the efficacy of coronary bypass surgery—II. *Am. J. Cardiol.,* 42:161–162.
16. Braunwald, E., and Maroko, P. R. (1974): The reduction of infarct size—An idea whose time (for testing) has come. *Circulation,* 50:206–209.
17. Bryson, A. L., Aycock, A. C., Flamm, M. D., Zaret, B. L., Ratshin, R. A., and McGowan, R. L. (1974): Changes in regional ventricular contraction of arteriosclerotic heart following nitroglycerin administration—Surgical correlation. *Circulation (Suppl. III),* 49/50:III-44 (abstr.).
18. Büll, U., Strauer, B. E., and Hast, B. (1976): Die 201-Thallium-Szintigraphie des Herzens als neues Verfahren zur Funktionellen Differenzierung der koronaren Herzkrankheit. *God. Zb. Med. Fak. Skopje,* 124:434–443.
19. Bussmann, W. D., Schöfer, H., and Kaltenbach, M. (1976): Wirkung von Nitroglycerin beim akuten Myokardinfarkt. II. Intravenöse Dauerinfusion von Nitroglycerin bei Patienten mit und ohne Linksinsuffizienz und ihre Auswirkungen auf die Infarktgrosse. *Dtsch. Med. Wochenschr.,* 101:642–648.
20. Cannom, D. S., Miller, D. C., Shumway, N. E., Fogarty, T. J., Daily, P. O., Hu, M., Brown, B., Jr., and Harrison, D. C. (1974): The long-term follow-up of patients undergoing saphenous vein bypass surgery. *Circulation,* 49:77–85.
21. Chatterjee, K., Matloff, J. M., Swan, H. J. C., Ganz, W., Kaushik, V. S., Magnusson, P., Henis, M. M., and Forrester, J. S. (1975): Abnormal regional metabolism and mechanical function in patients with ischemic heart disease; improvement after successful regional revascularization by aortocoronary bypass. *Circulation,* 52:390–399.
22. Chatterjee, K., Swan, H. J., Parmley, W. W., Sustaita, H., Marcus, H., and Matloff, J. (1972): Depression of left ventricular function due to acute myocardial ischemia and its reversal after aortocoronary saphenous-vein bypass. *N. Engl. J. Med.,* 286:1117–1122.
23. Chesebro, J. H., Ritman, E. L., Frye, R. L., Smith, H. C., Rutherford, B. D., Fulton, R. E., Pluth, J. R., and Barnhorst, D. A. (1978): Regional myocardial wall thickening response to nitroglycerin. A predictor of myocardial response to aortocoronary bypass surgery. *Circulation,* 57:952–957.
24. Cobb, L. A., Thomas, G. I., Dillard, D. H., Merendino, K. A., and Bruce, R. A. (1959): An evaluation of internal mammary artery ligation by a double blind technique. *N. Engl. J. Med.,* 260:1115–1118.
25. Come, P. C., Flaherty, J. T., Baird, M. G., Rouleau, J. R., Weisfeldt, M. L., Greene, H. L., Becker, L., and Pitt, B. (1975): Reversal by phenylephrine of the beneficial effects of intravenous nitroglycerin—Patients with acute myocardial infarction. *N. Engl. J. Med.,* 293:1003–1007.
26. Dodek, A., Kassebaum, D. G., and Griswold, H. E. (1973): Stress electrocardiography in the evaluation of aortocoronary bypass surgery. *Am. Heart J.,* 86:292–307.

27. Dunkman, W. B., Perloff, J. K., Kastor, J. A., and Shelburne, J. S. (1974): Medical perspectives in coronary artery surgery—A caveat. *Ann. Intern. Med.,* 81:817–837.
28. Dyke, S. H., Cohn, P. F., Gorlin, R., and Sonnenblick, E. H. (1974): Detection of residual myocardial function in coronary artery disease using post-extra systolic potentiation. *Circulation,* 50:694–699.
29. Effler, D. B., Favaloro, R. G., and Groves, L. K. (1970): Coronary artery surgery utilizing saphenous vein graft techniques. Clinical experience with 224 operations. *J. Thorac. Cardiovasc. Surg.,* 59:147–154.
30. Fischer-Hansen, J. E., and Sande, E. (1979): Prinzmetal's angina, coronary spasm. *Eur. J. Cardiol. (in press).*
31. Ganz, W., Tamura, K., Marcus, H. S., Donoso, R., Yoshida, S., and Swan, H. J. C. (1971): Measurement of coronary sinus blood flow by continuous thermodilution in man. *Circulation,* 44:181–195.
32. Gudbjarnason, S. (1972): The use of glycolytic metabolism in the assessment of hypoxia in human hearts. *Cardiology,* 57:35–46.
33. Hardarson, T., Henning, H., O'Rourke, R. A., Karliner, J. S., Ryan, W., and Ross, J., Jr. (1978): Variability, reproducibility and applications of precordial ST-segment mapping following acute myocardial infarction. *Circulation,* 57:1096–1103.
34. Helfant, R. H., Pine, R., Meister, S. G., Feldman, M. S., Trout, R. G., and Banka, V. S. (1974): Nitroglycerin to unmask reversible asynergy: Correlation with post coronary bypass ventriculography. *Circulation,* 50:108–113.
35. Jackson, G., Atkinson, L., and Oram, S. (1977): Improvement of myocardial metabolism in coronary arterial disease by beta-blockade. *Br. Heart J.,* 39:829–833.
36. Johnson, W. D., and Lepley, D., Jr. (1970): An aggressive surgical approach to coronary disease. *J. Thorac. Cardiovasc. Surg.,* 59:128–138.
37. de Jong, J. W., and Goldstein, S. (1974): Changes in coronary venous inosine concentration and myocardial wall thickening during regional ischemia in the pig. *Circ. Res.,* 35:111–116.
38. Kent, K. M., Borer, J. S., Green, M. V., Bacharach, St. L., McIntosh, C. L., Conkle, D. M., and Epstein, St. E. (1978): Effects of coronary-artery bypass on global and regional left ventricular function during exercise. *N. Engl. J. Med.,* 298:1434–1439.
39. Klausner, S. C., Ratshin, R. A., Tyberg, J. V., Lappin, H. A., Chatterjee, K., and Parmley, W. W. (1976): The similarity of changes in segmental contraction patterns induced by postextra-systolic potentiation and nitroglycerin. *Circulation,* 54:615–623.
40. Korbuly, D. E., Formanek, A., Gypser, G., Moore, R., Ovitt, T. W., Tuna, N., and Amplatz, K. (1975): Regional myocardial blood flow measurements before and after coronary bypass surgery. A preliminary report. *Circulation,* 52:38–45.
41. Kronenberg, M. W., Hodges, M., Akiyama, T., Roberts, D. L., Ehrich, D. A., Bidie, T. L., and Yu, P. N. (1976): ST-segment variations after acute myocardial infarction. Relationship to clinical status. *Circulation,* 54:756–765.
42. Kübler, W. (1974): Myocardial energy metabolism in patients with ischemic heart disease. *Basic Res. Cardiol.,* 69:105–112 (editorial).
43. Kugler, G. (1978): Myocardial release of lactate, inosine and hypoxanthine during atrial pacing and exercise-induced angina. *Circulation,* 59:43–49.
44. Kupper, W., and Bleifeld, W. (1979): Serum enzyme changes in patients with cardiac disease, *Adv. Clin. Enzymol.,* pp. 106–123.
45. Kupper, W., Bleifeld, W., and Hanrath, P. (1976): Great cardiac vein flow and regional myocardial metabolism in patients with isolated LAD-stenosis. *Circulation (Suppl. II),* 53/54:II-7.
46. Kupper, W., Bleifeld, W., Hanrath, P., and Essen, R. (1977): Precordial mapping in early myocardial infarction. In: *The First 24 Hours in Myocardial Infarction,* pp. 86–88. G. Witzstrock, Baden-Baden.
47. Kupper, W., Hanrath, P., Bleifeld, W., Vebis, R., and Effert, S. (1977): Natrium-nitroprussid zur Therapie der Linksinsuffizienz beim akuten Herzinfarkt. *Dtsch. Med. Wochenschr.,* 102:548–554.
48. Lee, S. J. K., Sung, K., and Zaragoza, A. J. (1970): Effects of nitroglycerin on left ventricular volumes and wall tension in patients with ischemic heart disease. *Br. Heart J.,* 32:790–794.
49. Lepley, D., Jr. (1972): Optimal resources of coronary artery surgery. Report of the Inter-Society Commission for Heart Disease Resources. *Ann. Thorac. Surg.,* 14:413–433.
50. Levine, J. A., Bechtel, D. J., Cohn, P. F., Herman, M. V., Gorlin, R., Cohn, L. H., and Collins, J. J., Jr. (1975): Ventricular function before and after direct revascularization surgery.

A proposal for an index of revascularization to correlate angiographic and ventriculographic findings. *Circulation,* 51:1071–1078.

51. Lichtlen, P. R., Engel, H.-J., and Hundeshagen, (n.i.) (1977): Regional myocardial blood flow in normal and poststenotic areas after nitroglycerin, beta-blockade (Atenolol), coronary dilatation. *Herz,* 2:81–86.

52. da Luz, P. L., Forrester, J. S., Wyatt, H. L., Tyberg, J. V., Chagrasulis, R., Parmley, W. W., and Swan, H. J. C. (1975): Hemodynamic and metabolic effects of sodium nitroprusside on the performance and metabolism of regional ischemic myocardium. *Circulation,* 52:400–407.

53. Di Luzio, V., Roy, P. R., and Sowton, E. (1974): Angina in patients with occluded aorto-coronary vein grafts. *Br. Heart J.,* 36:139–147.

54. Mann, T., Cohn, P. F., Holman, L. B., Green, L. H., Markis, J. E., and Phillips, D. A. (1978): Effect of nitroprusside on regional myocardial blood flow in coronary artery disease. Results in 25 patients and comparison with nitroglycerin. *Circulation,* 57:732–738.

55. Maroko, P. R., Kjekshus, J. K., Sobel, B. E., Watanabe, T., Covell, J. W., Ross, J., Jr., and Braunwald, E. (1971): Factors influencing infarct size following experimental coronary artery occlusions. *Circulation,* 43:67–82.

56. Maroko, P. R., Libby, P., Bloor, C. M., Sobel, B. E., Braunwald, E. (1972): Reduction by hyaluronidase of myocardial necrosis following coronary artery occlusion. *Circulation,* 46:430–437.

57. Maseri, A., Marzilli, M., Parodi, O., Severi, S., and L'Abbate, A. (1977): Regional myocardial perfusion in angina caused by increased demand in presence of critical coronary stenosis and in primary angina at rest. *Herz,* 2:65–69.

58. Mathey, D. (1977): Regionale mechanische und metabolische verändrangen bei graduierter myokardischämie. *Herz/Kreislauf,* 9:250–57.

59. Mathey, D., Bleifeld, W., Buss, H., and Hanrath, P. (1975): Creatine kinase release—acute myocardial information: Correlation with clinical, electrographic, and pathological findings. *Br. Heart J.,* 37:1161–1168.

60. Mathey, D., Bleifeld, W., Hanrath, P., and Effert, S. (1974): Attempt to quantitate relation between cardiac function and infarct size in acute myocardial infarction. *Br. Heart J.,* 36:271–279.

61. Mathey, D., Montz, R., Hanrath, P., Knop, J., Kupper, W., Schneider, C., and Bleifeld, W. (1978): Kurzfristige regionale myokardischaemie und ihre folgen bei prinzmetal-angina pectoris. *Dtsch. Med. Wochenschr.,* 103:968–971.

62. Mathey, D., Montz, R., Hanrath, P., Kupper, W., Bleese, N., Vorbringer, H., and Bleifeld, W. (1978): Reversible Myokardischaemie oder Irreversible Myokardfibrose? Untersuchung mit Hilfe der biphasischen 201-Thallium-Szintigraphie. *Dtsch. Med. Wochenschr.,* 103:1736–1739.

63. Merrill, A. J., Jr., Thomas, C., Schechter, E., Cline, R., Armstrong, R., and Stanford, W. (1975): Coronary bypass surgery; value of maximal exercise testing in assessment of results. *Circulation (Suppl. I),* 51/52:I-173–I-177.

64. Miller, D. W., Jr., Bruce, R. A., and Dodge, H. T. (1978): Physiologic improvement following coronary artery bypass surgery. *Circulation,* 57:831–835.

65. Miller, J. E., Maroko, P. R., and Braunwald, E. (1975): Evaluation of precordial electrocardiographic mapping as a means of assessing changes in myocardial injury. *Circulation,* 52:16–27.

66. Mills, R. M., Young, E., Gorlin, R., and Lesch, M. (1975): Natural history of S-T segment elevation after acute myocardial infarction. *Am. J. Cardiol.,* 35:609–614.

67. Miura, M., Ganz, W., Thomas, R., Singh, B. N., Sokol, T., and Shell, W. E. (1976): Reduction of infarct size by propranolol in closed-chest anesthetized dogs. *Circulation (Suppl. II),* 53/54:II-159 (Abstr.).

68. Norris, R. M., Whitlock, R. M. L., Barratt-Boyes, C., and Small, C. W. (1975): Clinical measurement of myocardial infarct size. Modification of a method for the estimation of total creatine phosphokinase release after myocardial infarction. *Circulation,* 51:614–620.

69. Opie, L. H. (1971): Substrate utilization and glycolysis in the heart. *Cardiology,* 56:2–21.

70. Opie, L. H., Owen, P., Thomas, M., and Samson, R. (1973): Coronary sinus lactate measurements in assessment of myocardial ischemia. *Am. J. Cardiol.,* 32:295–305.

71. Pachinger, O., Probst, P., Ogris, E., and Kaindl, F. (1977): Quantitative scintigraphic imaging in myocardium using TL-201 in patients with coronary heart-disease. *Herz/Kreislauf,* 9:310–315.

72. Page, D. L., Caulfield, J. B., Kastor, J. A., DeSanctis, R. W., and Sanders, C. A. (1971): Myocardial changes associated with cardiogenic shock. *N. Engl. J. Med.,* 285:133–137.

73. Parker, J. O., West, R. O., Case, R. B., and Chiong, M. A. (1969): Temporal relationships of myocardial lactate metabolism, left ventricular function, and ST-segment depression during angina precipitated by exercise. *Circulation,* 40:97–111.
74. Parmley, W. W., Chatterjee, K., Charuzi, Y., and Swan, H. J. C. (1974): Hemodynamic effects of noninvasive systolic unloading (nitroprusside) and diastolic augmentation (external counter-pulsation) in patients with acute myocardial infarction. *Am. J. Cardiol.,* 33:819–825.
75. Peter, T., Norris, R. M., Clarke, E. D., Heng, M. K., Singh, B. N., Williams, B., Howell, D. R., and Ambler, P. K. (1978): Reduction of enzyme levels by propranolol after acute myocardial infarction. *Circulation,* 57:1091–1095.
76. Reid, D. S., Pelides, L. J., and Shillingford, J. P. (1971): Surface mapping of RS-T segment in acute myocardial infarction. *Br. Heart J.,* 33:370–374.
77. Reid, P. R., Taylor, D. R., Kelly, D. T., Wiesfelt, M. L., Humphries, J. O., Ross, R. S., and Pitt, B. (1974): Myocardial-infarct extension detected by precordial ST-segment mapping. *N. Engl. J. Med.,* 290:123–128.
78. Ritchie, J. L., Hamilton, G. W., and Wackers, F. J. Th. (1978): *Thallium-201 Myocardial Imaging.* Raven Press, New York.
79. Ritchie, J. L., Narahara, K. A., Trobaugh, G. B., Williams, D. L. and Hamilton, G. W. (1977): Thallium-201 myocardial imaging before and after coronary revascularization: Assessment of regional myocardial blood flow and graft patency. *Circulation,* 56:830–836.
80. Roberts, R., Husain, A., Ambos, H. D., Oliver, G. C., Cox, J. R., Jr., and Sobel, B. E. (1975): Relation between infarct size and ventricular arrhythmia. *Br. Heart J.,* 37:1169–1175.
81. Robinson, C., Jackson, G., Fisk, C., and Jewitt, D. (1978): Haemodynamic effects of atenolol in patients with coronary artery disease. *Br. Heart J.,* 40:22–28.
82. Rogers, W. J., McDaniel, H. G., Smith, L. R., Mantlem, J. A., Russel, R. O., and Rackley, C. E. (1977): Correlation of angiographic estimates of myocardial infarct size and accumulated release of creatine kinase MB isoenzyme in man. *Circulation,* 56:199–205.
83. Ross, R. S. (1975): Ischemic heart disease: An overview. *Am. J. Cardiol.,* 36:496–505.
84. Selwyn, A. P., Fox, K., Welman, E., and Shillingford, J. P. (1978): Natural history and evaluation of Q waves during acute myocardial infarction. *Br. Heart J.,* 40:383–387.
85. Selwyn, A. P., Ogunro, E. A., and Shillingford, J. P. (1977): Natural history and evaluation of ST segment changes and MB CK release in acute myocardial infarction. *Br. Heart J.,* 39:988–994.
86. Shell, W. E., and Sobel, B. E. (1973): Prediction of infarct size from serum CPK changes early after myocardial infarction. *Am. J. Cardiol.,* 31:157L (Abstr.).
87. Shell, W. E., and Sobel, B. E. (1974): Protection of jeopardized ischemic myocardium by reduction of ventricular afterload. *N. Engl. J. Med.,* 291:481–486.
88. Sobel, B. E., Bresnahan, G. F., Shell, W. E., and Yoder, R. D. (1972): Estimation of infarct size in man and its relation to prognosis. *Circulation,* 46:640–648.
89. Strauss, H. W., and Pitt, B. (1978): Evaluation of cardiac function and structure with radioactive tracer techniques. *Circulation,* 57:645–654.
90. Tennant, R., and Wiggers, C. J. (1935): Effect of coronary occlusion on myocardial contraction. *Am. J. Physiol.,* 112:351–361.
91. Varonkov, Y., Shell, W., Smirnov, V., and Chazov, E. (1975): Augmentation of CPK-infarct size by digitalis. *Circulation (Suppl. II),* 51/52:II-107 (Abstr.).
92. Wolf, R., Habel, F., Beckers, G., Krauss, H., and Lichtlen, P. (1978): Beziehung zwischen enzymchemisch und angiographisch bestimmter Infarktgrosse des linken Ventrikels. *Z. Kardiol.,* 67:225 (Abstract).

Ischemic Myocardium and Antianginal Drugs,
edited by M. M. Winbury and Y. Abiko.
Raven Press, New York © 1979.

Discussion: Myocardial Blood Flow

Wolfgang Schaper, *Chairman*

W. Schaper: An enormous amount of material has been presented during this session, and I will exercise my privilege as chairman to ask the first question of Dr. Winbury. You stated that reserve in the endocardium is much less than in the epicardium. I would go along with this view. However, one has to bear in mind two important factors. First, the myocardial oxygen consumption under which experiments have been carried out should be considered. You have repeatedly said that you reduced flow so and so much percent from normal flow. Now normal flow can scatter widely in the heart depending on the actual oxygen consumption. This is point one. And I think that the other very important point is that one has to define the extravascular factors because these play a very important role in the subendocardial blood flow. Would you like to comment on these two questions?

Winbury: With regard to myocardial oxygen consumption, we actually have no measurement of what happens to MVo_2 when we reduce flow. In line with Dr. Opie's comment, Gregg suggested that oxygen consumption was flow dependent, but this is not universally accepted. The one thing that possibly saves us to some extent is that Po_2 depends on the relationship between MVo_2 and the oxygen supply. Our primary objective was to produce maximal vasodilatation in each region. This would vary depending on oxygen consumption. With respect to the second point about the extravascular factors, I think you are referring primarily to wall tension. That is another factor that we did not take into account and that will affect the subendocardium. As we reduce flow, the compliance is going to be diminished to some extent. Those two factors come into play, and there is no simple way of getting around them.

W. Schaper: Thank you. Are there related questions?

Opie: On the question of the myocardial oxygen tension difference between the endocardial and epicardial, you did not stress this in your presentation. You have, of course, very frequently been quoted in relation to your nitroglycerin results, which as I recall indicate an increase in the endocardial oxygen tension. Now this would suggest a local effect of nitroglycerin. I wonder if this is a very important point, one that we might like to discuss in principle. Furthermore, I wonder if it goes against Dr. Bleifeld's observations and his conclusion that it is a peripheral phenomenon, at least in his patients with severe coronary artery stenosis. So how do you feel about the local versus general effect of nitroglycerin?

Winbury: I do not think my findings are contrary to what Dr. Bleifeld has said. There is a recent paper by one of my former co-workers, Dr. Weiss, in which oxygen consumption in both regions of the heart was measured by a microspectrophotometric technique; his findings confirmed our theoretically predicted 20% higher oxygen consumption in subendocardium. He also showed *(unpublished data)* that nitroglycerin produces a greater diminution of oxygen consumption in the subendocardium. Now this may or may not be a direct effect, but the peripheral effects come into play; that is, reducing the preload reduces work of the subendocardium to a greater extent than that of the subepicardium because of the differences in fiber length. Fibers are longer in the subendocardium than in the subepicardium, and they contract to a greater extent. So with a smaller left ventricular volume, there will be a greater oxygen saving in a deep region. In addition, if we are correct about redistribution of flow by nitroglycerin, which we showed with the Po_2 as well as with perfusion, then although total coronary flow will not be changed, the distribution of flow will be altered, favoring a distribution toward the ischemic region or toward the subendocardium in that particular circumstance. Does that answer your question?

Opie: Yes. And how does Dr. Bleifeld feel about that?

W. Schaper: May we first hear from Dr. Bing on this very interesting question of whether nitroglycerin works directly on the heart or redistributes volumes?

Bing: Dr. Winbury, you mentioned that inflow in the subendocardium is greatest during diastole, did you not?

Winbury: That's right.

Bing: Well, I think this is certainly true when you look at the flow in the arterioles. I just want to say again that when you look at the capillaries, the greatest amount of flow, whether it's subendocardial or subepicardial, occurs during systole. One has to make a sharp distinction. We have taken movie after movie and demonstrated that there is a 180° turn between arterial or arteriolar and capillary flow. I think, however, that Dr. Schaper was right when he started to mention wall tension in this situation. When you look at the films, the capillaries are squeezed out at tremendous rate by the contraction. I think that nitroglycerin will make a change in the subendocardium, and the passage time during systole will become longer.

Winbury: I think you are right here. There is a recent review by Julian Hoffman that discusses the emptying of blood vessels during systole and the refilling during diastole so that there would be flow during both phases of the cardiac cycle. I agree that capillary flow would be continued, but would the flow be adequate to maintain metabolism during systole?

W. Schaper: Let us hear Dr. Bleifeld's view on nitroglycerin, and then I suggest we go to a different topic.

Bleifeld: The only thing I could argue is that the methods we used cannot really answer this question. I would like to mention the studies of Ganz, who injected nitroglycerin directly in the coronary artery. He did not get any effect on angina, although he saw, in some patients, an increase in flow.

W. Schaper: Well, thank you. Dr. Hashimoto.

Hashimoto: I got a heart attack 11 years ago. I do not think the endocardial portion is more important than the epicardial for cardiac function. Can you tell me what part is the most important for cardiac function?

Winbury: I really cannot answer because both parts contribute to function.

Hashimoto: Same importance?

W. Schaper: Is there any volunteer to answer that?

Bing: I do not think you can get along with one without the other.

Nakamura: I would like to ask you, Dr. Winbury, about factors contributing to the vulnerability of the subendocardium compared to the subepicardium. In the control state, diastolic flow is a major supply to the endocardium. However, if you produce stenosis, the percentage of contributing flow in systole increases. Do you count this in the vulnerability of the subendocardium?

Winbury: That was also considered in the paper by Julian Hoffman. He showed that, as one increases stenosis, the proportionality changes and the diastole/systole flow ratio decreases from 4 to 1 almost 1 to 1. Ultimately, there is no perfusion of the deep region. For that reason, I was interested in measuring perfusion pressure and the critical closing pressure because these give us some index of when the wall tension causes complete collapse in those regions. So it is a matter of diastolic perfusion pressure and diastolic perfusion time that is relevant to the supply to the endocardium.

W. Schaper: Well, thank you very much. I think that answers most of Dr. Nakamura's question. I hope you will forgive me if I propose to go to a different topic and ask Dr. Hashimoto about the different sensitivities among the vascular beds and among the drugs he has studied. Is it possible that these differences could be attributed in part to coronary arteries that have a very high degree of reserve, that is, arteries that can increase the amount of flow four- to sixfold, depending on initial oxygen consumption? Let us take, for example, the renal artery, which is a high-flow artery to begin with. Could this somehow enter into the picture and explain, in part, the differences in sensitivity that you've found, Dr. Hashimoto?

Hashimoto: This is a tricky business to make such a conclusion from our data, which was presented only in percentage increase. Another point is that the preparation was perfused with blood at a constant pressure of 100 mm Hg, but responses of the femoral and coronary arteries may be different because the skeletal muscle that the femoral artery supplies with blood is in a state of rest while the heart is in an active state. So it is not fair to compare the response of the femoral artery to that of the coronary artery.

W. Schaper: I hope you will forgive me if I pursue the question further. Have you or has anyone in the audience any idea how much the renal flow can increase? What is the maximal flow? Is it 100, 200, or 300%?

Nakamura: Renal blood flow depends on the perfusion pressure in this case. Normally, the blood flow is autoregulated. But when the calcium antagonists are administered, the renal vessels lose their autoregulation. Therefore the sensitivity of vasodilatation must be considered in relation to the perfusion pressure.

W. Schaper: Sure, but I think one of the definitions of autoregulation is its independence of the perfusion pressure. Autoregulation, as I understand, is a curve that goes up, shows a plateau, and then goes up again. Now if you measure it in the physiological range, the flow stays constant while you increase the pressure. Therefore, you cannot say that it is pressure dependent.

Opie: Mr. Chairman, may I join you in your confusion on a different subject. Would somebody, possibly Dr. Hashimoto, define for us clearly what we mean by a calcium-antagonistic drug. Dr. Bing said that there have been 10 mechanisms proposed at Tokyo of which he only understood two. I only understood one. Is it perhaps not controversial to include perhexiline as a calcium-antagonistic drug?

Hashimoto: This is a very good question. Professor Fleckenstein is a good friend of mine, but I have never agreed with him that perhexiline is a calcium-antagonistic drug. His preparation of the ventricular muscle is from guinea pigs and aortic strips from pigs. So, it is quite difficult to make a conclusion, I have wondered whether perhexiline should be included in the calcium-antagonistic drugs and have relied only on his definition.

Bing: To quote the Pope himself, I mean Dr. Fleckenstein, by definition his paper says that these are substances that inhibit movement of calcium within the cell without inhibiting sodium and potassium movement. In other words, this is where the electromechanical dissociation comes from because mechanical function diminishes, primarily as a result of the effect on the sarcolemma, whereas sodium and potassium ATPase are not disturbed. Dr. Fleckenstein's is a good definition.

Henry: However, if I am not mistaken, electrophysiologists have demonstrated that verapamil and diltiazem may also exert inhibitory effects on the sodium channel. The importance of the local anesthetic effects of these drugs will require further evaluation.

Hashimoto: Diltiazem is very similar to verapamil in our preparation, so diltiazem is close to verapamil and can be classified as a calcium-antagonistic drug.

W. Schaper: I think that the simplest definition of the calcium antagonist is that whatever effect the drug produces can be reversed by adding calcium. Is this correct?

Henry: There are many negative inotropic interventions that can be partly transiently overcome with calcium, such as ischemia, for instance. You are not going to call ischemia a calcium antagonist. I think the reversal by calcium is a very nonspecific effect. There is the stimulatory effect of calcium during a number of negative inotropic interventions.

W. Schaper: Yes, that is true, and I remember Dr. Fleckenstein saying that nitroglycerin is a calcium antagonist.

Henry: Yes, that is quite correct. It is correct to say that the calcium antagonists inhibit the slow inward movement in certain voltage clamp experiments. However, it would be fair to investigate other drugs with the same technique at the same time and under the same experimental condition. In fact, I think it would be essential.

W. Schaper: Thank you. Any comment?

Winbury: I think one of the interesting points of Dr. Bleifeld's presentation is the effect of cardiac bypass surgery. The increase in the reserve in some of the patients would indicate that you have improved distal perfusion and have increased the perfusion area. Yet there is still controversy about the effect of bypass surgery on perfusion. Your study certainly does show that there was an increase in the reserve under atrial stimulation. Do I interpret that correctly?

Bleifeld: Yes, but my conclusion was that in some patients we do not see this. The problem is that some patients do not have angina afterwards. So, from the history, you cannot evaluate the effect of the surgery.

Winbury: You mean you cannot evaluate why the patient has improved? Is that what you are saying? You said angina may disappear in those in which you did not increase the reserve.

Bleifeld: In some, yes. You definitely can increase the flow.

Bing: I would like to remind you of experiments done many years ago before the coronary artery bypass operation was invented. One simply ligated the internal mammary artery, and people improved considerably. We all have something upstairs, as well as down here.

Bleifeld: I would like to add one comment. The main problem is not only to prove that coronary bypass surgery has an effect but to look for the ideal candidate beforehand.

W. Schaper: I would like to ask Dr. Bing about his wonderful result with this new drug, diltiazem, and I would like to know if all these favorable responses are somehow linked to the metabolic state of the heart in a more general way. That is, does diltiazem reduce the myocardial oxygen requirement to such a degree that this would be a common denominator to all the metabolic things that you have measured?

Bing: I do not think that a reduction in oxygen requirement is the common denominator. Nitroglycerin and molsidomin produce a diminution of the oxygen requirement of the heart but nothing at all as far as respiration of mitochondria is concerned, and calcium uptake and binding are completely unchanged. I do not think this is the common requirement. It would be very nice if such a baseline could be found. But I do not understand the effect of this drug.

W. Schaper: Yes. May I pursue this question? You have just mentioned the oxygen requirement under nitroglycerin and molsidomin, but I remember one of your slides showed a diminution of oxygen consumption from an average value of 11 ml to an average value of 9 ml.

Bing: This is the effect of molsidomin and was quoted from Germany.

W. Schaper: This is not extremely striking. I mean, when you infuse, let's say, a morphine derivative that slows the heart rate, you can arrive at an MVo_2 of about 5 ml/min/100 g. This probably produces a very profound metabolic effect.

Bing: Although the effect of molsidomin may be modest, with nitroglycerin, they found very marked diminution in the oxygen consumption of the myocardium, again without metabolic changes.

W. Schaper: Is there any comment?

Bing: May I make one general comment? We are looking at the effect of antianginal drugs on metabolism and hemodynamics. I just want to say something as a clinician. Very often, we find a marked dissociation between what the mitochondria are doing and what the patient does. That's the impression I have often received. I think this is a serious comment because the mitochondria may be improved in a patient who feels worse, and the forward load or backward load may diminish and yet no effect becomes apparent.

W. Schaper: Thank you very much.

Hashimoto: May I comment on molsidomin? Molsidomin itself does not show any effect on cardiac function. In my preparation, only propranolol reduced it.

Bing: Well, I think you are right, but it depends on what you understand cardiac function to be. Molsidomin does not change metabolic function. On the other hand, it does seem to cause a redistribution of blood. Nitroglycerin does a very similar thing. The only difference between the two is that molsidomin lasts 5 hr and gives more of a headache, and nitroglycerin lasts only 20 min. So I just want to say again that there are ways to reach nirvana, and I think molsidomin may be one of them.

W. Schaper: Well, thank you very much for your discussion.

Antianginal Drugs

Ischemic Myocardium and Antianginal Drugs,
edited by M. M. Winbury and Y. Abiko.
Raven Press, New York © 1979.

Effects of Diltiazem, a New Antianginal Drug, on Myocardial Blood Flow Following Experimental Coronary Occlusion

Motoomi Nakamura, Yasushi Koiwaya, Akira Yamada, Yutaka Kikuchi, Yutaka Senda, Tomihiro Ikeo, Kenji Sunagawa, Michitaka Mori, and Hideo Kanaide

Research Institute of Angiocardiology and Cardiovascular Clinic, Kyushu University Medical School, Fukuoka 812, Japan

Since myocardial ischemia associated with coronary occlusive disease results from an imbalance between myocardial oxygen demand and supply, drug therapy designed to reduce ischemia and infarct size must produce restoration of the balance in the ischemic myocardium through either augmentation in myocardial blood flow or a diminution of oxygen consumption (1). The validity of the concept that ischemic injury can be reduced by diverse pharmacologic interventions has been demonstrated (4). It has been demonstrated that collateral flow usually starts to increase approximately 6 to 24 hr after an acute coronary occlusion in dogs (13). Oxygen supply to the ischemic area in dogs with complete coronary occlusion is dependent on collateral circulation, and dilatation of the collateral vessels may increase blood flow to the ischemic area. This chapter summarizes studies on effects of a new calcium antagonist, diltiazem—d-3-acetoxy-cis-2,3-dihydro-5-[2-(dimethylamino)ethyl]-2-(p-methoxyphenyl)1,5-benzothiazepine-4(5H)-1-hydrochloride—that has been used as an antianginal agent in man (19) and is known to dilate the collateral vessel (6) in myocardial ischemia following coronary occlusion.

MATERIALS AND METHODS

Experimental Myocardial Infarction

Experiment 1 (Open-Chest Dogs)

Effects of diltiazem on *myocardial ischemia following acute coronary artery occlusion* [*experiment I*(a)] were studied in 19 mongrel dogs of either sex (weight 12 to 27 kg) under open chest and anesthesia with chloralose and urethane. Respiration was maintained mechanically with a Harvard respirator. The heart

129

was exposed by thoracotomy, and the left anterior descending coronary artery (LAD) distal to the first diagonal branch was ligated completely using a two-step technique. Epicardial electrocardiograms (EKGs) were recorded from three sites on the ischemic, three sites on the border, and three sites on the nonischemic area of the left ventricle. Catheters were placed in the aorta to measure blood pressure and obtain a reference sample, in the left atrium to inject tracer microspheres and measure pressure, and in the vein to inject diltiazem or saline solution. Three different tracer microspheres (^{46}Sc, ^{85}Sr, and ^{141}Ce) were injected before and 30 min after LAD occlusion and 1.5 min after intravenous injection of saline (0.2 ml/kg) or diltiazem HCl (100 μg/kg) for 20 sec, as shown in Fig. 1. Animals were divided into two groups receiving saline (8 dogs) and diltiazem (11 dogs). The heart was removed 30 min after drug or saline, and regional myocardial blood flow was measured as described below.

Studies on myocardial blood flow in dogs with chronic myocardial infarction [experiment 1(b)] were performed in eight mongrel dogs (weight 10 to 15 kg) under open chest and anesthesia with chloralose and urethane. The experimental procedure to produce acute myocardial infarction by LAD occlusion was identical with that described above in experiment 1(a), except for an aseptic condition, and the first tracer microspheres were injected 30 min after LAD occlusion (Fig. 1). The chest was then closed, and 3 to 5 weeks after LAD occlusion, the heart was reexposed and the second tracer microspheres were injected into the left atrium. One and one-half minutes after injection of diltiazem (100 μg/kg) taking 20 sec, the third tracer microspheres were injected. After removing

Experiment I (open-chest)

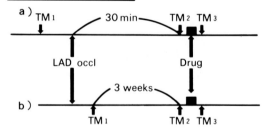

Experiment II (conscious)

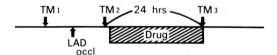

FIG. 1. Experimental schedule for experiments 1(a,b) and 2. TM, tracer microspheres; LAD, left anterior descending coronary artery; Drug, diltiazem or saline; occl, occlusion.

the heart, regional blood flow of the left ventricular free wall was measured as described below.

Experiment 2 (Conscious Dogs)

Sixteen beagle dogs weighing 7 to 13 kg were divided into two groups: the control group (seven dogs) and the diltiazem group (nine dogs). In both groups the LAD distal to the first diagonal branch was freed and equipped with an occluder during an aseptic operation. Catheters were placed into the ascending aorta for measurement of arterial blood pressure, the femoral vein for injection of the drug, and the left atrium for the injection of the tracer microspheres. All catheters were exteriorized and secured in the skin between the scapulae. The animals were allowed to recover and received antibiotics for 3 days. The catheters were filled with heparin. After return of serum creatine phosphokinase (CPK) to the preoperative level, LAD was acutely occluded by the occluder until the end of experiment. Arterial blood pressure and precordial electrocardiogram (EKG) were recorded until sacrifice. In the control group, saline was given intravenously for 24 hr after LAD occlusion. In the diltiazem group, 20 μg/kg/min of diltiazem for the first 15 min followed by 10 μg/kg/min of diltiazem for the remaining 23¾ hours were continuously infused intravenously. Three differently labeled tracer microspheres (^{85}Sr, ^{46}Sc, and ^{141}Ce) were injected before and 15 min and 24 hr after LAD occlusion (Fig. 1). After the injection of the third tracer microspheres (TM3), dogs were sacrificed and regional blood flow of the left ventricle was measured as described below.

Measurement of Regional Myocardial Blood Flow

Changes in regional myocardial blood flow were measured by the tracer microsphere technique as reported previously (9). Three differently labeled tracer microspheres, 15 μm in diameter in experiment 1 and 8 to 10 μm in diameter in experiment 2, were used in random sequence. For each determination, approximately 0.5 to 1×10^6 microspheres in experiment 1 and 4 to 8×10^6 microspheres in experiment 2 were injected, and the arterial blood reference sample was aspirated for 1.5 min. The left ventricular free wall was divided into 26 (experiment 2) or 36 (experiment 1) full-thickness sections, and each section was sliced further into subendocardial, middle, and subepicardial layers. Gamma spectrometry was carried out on these tissues and on reference blood samples with an automated nuclear data computer system as described previously (9).

Definition of Control and Ischemic Area

The myocardial segments located at the posterior area of the left ventricular free wall, which the left circumflex coronary artery supplied, were defined as a control area, weighing about 4 to 6 g. Myocardial blood flow (percentage) of each myocardial segment was related to the control area by radioactivity of the tracer microspheres injected 15 to 30 min after acute LAD occlusion. The segments of the left ventricular free wall were classified into nonischemic (> 75%), border (between 74 and 31%), and ischemic (< 30%) areas.

Measurement of ST Segment Elevation

In acute open-chest dogs [experiment 1(a)], the average ST segment elevation $[(\Sigma ST/N) = (\overline{ST})]$ at sites greater than 5 mV after occlusion was calculated as reported by Maroko et al. (5).

Determination of Infarct Size by Serum CPK

In experiment 2, determination of infarct size by the serum CPK was performed by the method described by Shell et al. (14). Serum CPK was measured 3, 5, 6, 7, 8, 9, 10, 11, 12, 13, 15, 18, 21, and 24 hr after coronary occlusion, and the best-fit curve was obtained by using the data observed from the entire duration of the experiment (i.e., 3 to 24 hr after coronary occlusion). The animals that died during the experimental period were excluded from the study.

RESULTS

Experiment 1 (Open-Chest Dogs and Short Period of Injection of Diltiazem)

Acute Myocardial Infarction

Ischemic ST Elevation

The effect of diltiazem treatment on average ST segment elevation $(\overline{ST})$ is summarized in Fig. 2. Average elevation of ST segment after intravenous injection of diltiazem (100 µg/kg) for 20 sec was significantly lower than that after saline injection (control group), which indicates that the severity of the myocardial injury was reduced by diltiazem injection.

Hemodynamics

Figure 3 demonstrates the effects of intravenous administration of diltiazem over 20 sec (100 µg/kg) on heart rate and on mean arterial and left atrial pressure. After diltiazem, heart rate and arterial blood pressure (mean, systolic, and diastolic) decreased significantly and returned gradually to the previous level. PR interval was prolonged transiently but significantly from 0.09 to 0.11 sec after diltiazem ($p < 0.01$) and returned to the previous level after 20 min. The left atrial pressure was not different in the two groups throughout the entire period, as shown in Fig. 3.

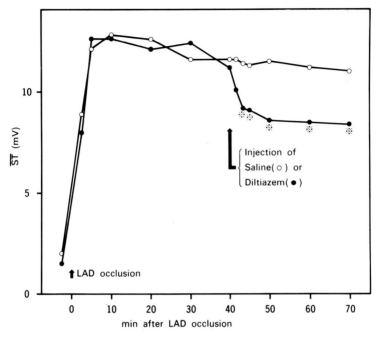

FIG. 2. Effect of diltiazem on epicardial $\overline{ST}$ [experiment 1(a)]. Average $\overline{ST}$ elevation in all sites at various times after occlusion in a control group *(open circles)* and a diltiazem group *(solid circles)*. *, Statistical significance between the two groups ($p < 0.01$).

Myocardial Blood Flow

Regional myocardial blood flow, as well as subendocardial to subepicardial flow ratio, decreased significantly after acute LAD occlusion in the ischemic area, but remained unchanged in the nonischemic area, as shown in Fig. 4. Intravenous administration of diltiazem (100 μg/kg for 20 sec) increased myocardial blood flow significantly in the nonischemic area of the left ventricle from about 1.1 ml/g/min to 2.0 ml/g/min ($p < 0.001$), but flow in the acutely ischemic area remained unchanged, as shown in Fig. 4.

Chronic Myocardial Infarction

Myocardial blood flow in the ischemic area increased significantly approximately 3 weeks after LAD occlusion, as compared with flow estimated from radioactivities of tracer microspheres injected 15 min after the LAD occlusion. This increase in flow was greater in the subepicardial layer than in the subendocardial layer. Diltiazem further increased myocardial blood flow, and the increase in flow after diltiazem was greater in the subepicardial layer of the ischemic area than in the subendocardial layer ($p < 0.05$), as shown in Fig. 5. In chronic

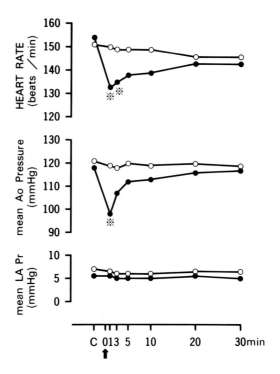

FIG. 3. Effects of diltiazem on hemodynamics. Diltiazem (100 µg/kg i.v.) was given for 20 sec *(arrow).* *, Significant difference between the control *(open circles)* and diltiazem *(solid circles)* groups ($p < 0.01$). Ao, aorta; LA Pr, left atrial pressure; C, before drug.

myocardial infarction, diltiazem increased flow but not the subendocardial/subepicardial flow ratio in the nonischemic area. A decrease in blood pressure and heart rate and prolongation of PR interval were also found after diltiazem, as in experiment 1(a).

Experiment 2 [Conscious Dog (Closed Chest) and Continuous Infusion of Diltiazem]

Hemodynamics

In conscious dogs, heart rate increased gradually after acute LAD occlusion (as shown in Fig. 6), but the heart rate of dogs receiving diltiazem was significantly lower 6 and 24 hr after LAD occlusion than that of the control dogs ($p < 0.05$ and $p < 0.01$, respectively). Mean blood pressure decreased gradually after LAD occlusion, but no significant difference in blood pressure was found between the control and diltiazem groups. Mean left atrial pressure in both groups increased transiently after LAD occlusion ($p < 0.05$), but no significant difference was found during the entire experimental period between the two

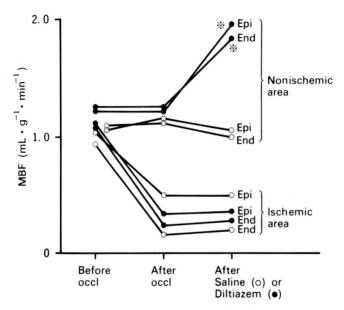

FIG. 4. Effects of diltiazem on myocardial blood flow (MBF; milliliters per gram per minute) of dogs with acute LAD occlusion (open chest). Diltiazem (100 μg/kg i.v.) was given for 20 sec. *, Significant difference between the control *(open circles)* and diltiazem *(solid circles)* groups ($p < 0.01$). Epi, subepicardial layer; End, subendocardial layer.

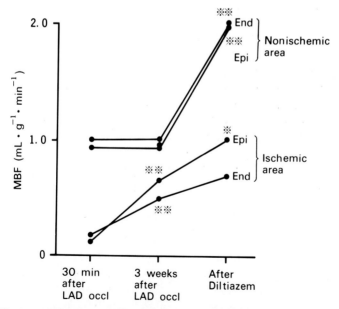

FIG. 5. Effects of diltiazem on MBF (milliliters per gram per minute) in chronic myocardial infarction (open chest). Diltiazem (100 μg/kg i.v.) was given for 20 sec. A statistical significance was found when MBF was compared with that in the previous stage (*, $p < 0.05$; **, $p < 0.01$).

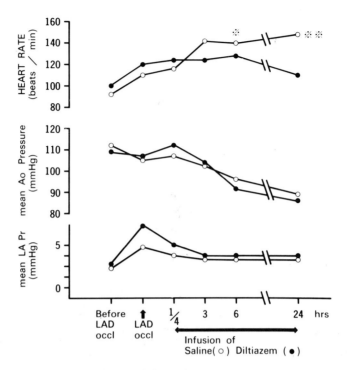

FIG. 6. Effects of continuous infusion of diltiazem on hemodynamics (conscious dogs). A statistically significant difference was found between the control *(open circles)* and diltiazem *(solid circles)* groups (*, $p < 0.05$; **, $p < 0.01$).

groups, as shown in Fig. 6. As in experiment 1(a,b), PR interval increased significantly from 0.11 to 0.13 ($p < 0.05$), but second degree atrioventricular block was not found during infusion of diltiazem. Frequent premature ventricular contraction began to occur consistently about 4 to 6 hr after occlusion and continued to the end of the experiment. Frequency of premature ventricular contraction in dogs receiving continuous infusion of diltiazem was significantly lower than that of the control group 22 and 24 hr after occlusion ($p < 0.01$ in both periods).

Myocardial Blood Flow

Changes of subendocardial and subepicardial blood flow in the nonischemic and ischemic areas are demonstrated in Fig. 7. Fifteen min after occlusion, blood flow in the nonischemic area remained unchanged in both groups. Diltiazem tended to increase subepicardial flow in the nonischemic area 24 hr after occlusion, but the increase was not statistically significant. Myocardial blood flow during the preocclusion period was about 15% lower in the ischemic area than in the nonischemic area, which suggests loss of microspheres from

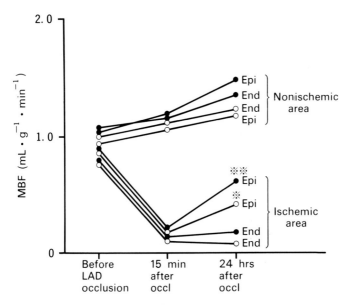

FIG. 7. Effects of continuous infusion of diltiazem on MBF (milliliters per gram per minute) in conscious dogs. A significant difference was found between MBF labeled * and ** ($p < 0.05$).

the necrotic myocardium. In the ischemic area, myocardial blood flow decreased 15 min after occlusion to about 15% of the preocclusion level in the subendocardium and 20% of the preocclusion level in the subepicardium in both groups. There was a significant increase in subepicardial blood flow to the ischemic tissue in both groups from 15 min to 24 hr after occlusion when compared with flow 15 min after occlusion ($p < 0.01$). However, this increase must be viewed cautiously because of microsphere loss (as described later). Subepicardial flow of the ischemic area 24 hr after LAD occlusion in the diltiazem group was significantly greater than in the control group ($p < 0.05$). The flow in the diltiazem group reached about 50 to 70% of preocclusion levels in the ischemic subepicardium by 24 hr, but did not increase in the ischemic subendocardium; thus the subendocardial/subepicardial flow ratio was decreased. In the border area, myocardial blood flow changed similarly to that in the ischemic area, but was less pronounced. The flow ratio of subendocardial to subepicardial layers in the nonischemic as well as ischemic areas was not significantly different between the two groups at all periods of the experimental schedule (i.e., before LAD occlusion and 15 min and 24 hr after LAD occlusion).

Effects of Diltiazem on Myocardial Infarct Size Estimated by Serial Serum CPK

The myocardial infarct size calculated from observed serum CPK changes was 14.5 ± 2.1 g (mean $\pm$ SE) and 15.4 ± 4.4 g in the control and diltiazem groups, respectively. The difference in the infarct size estimated by serum CPK changes between the two groups was not statistically significant. The relationship between infarct size estimated from serum CPK changes and ischemic area estimated from myocardial blood flow as an area less than 30% of the control area was poor and not statistically significant in both groups ($r = -0.23$ and $r = 0.42$ in the control and diltiazem groups, respectively).

DISCUSSION

Effect of Diltiazem on Myocardial Injury

Experiment 1(a) demonstrated that the treatment of acute myocardial infarction with diltiazem decreased the ST segment elevation significantly in epicardial recordings obtained in the early stage after acute coronary occlusion, which suggests a decrease in myocardial ischemic injury after diltiazem. Recently, experimental studies demonstrated that verapamil, a calcium antagonist, reduced ST segment elevation in dogs following acute coronary artery occlusion (17). However, an increase in collateral flow to the ischemic myocardium or a change in anaerobic metabolism was not associated with the reduction of ST segment elevation after verapamil, which suggests that verapamil reduces ischemic injury by direct myocardial effect (15). The reasons for the observed reduction in myocardial injury by diltiazem may be complex, and factors influencing dynamic balance between myocardial oxygen supply and demand must be considered. An increase in myocardial blood flow to the ischemic area was not found in experiment 1(a). A decrease in heart rate and arterial pressure can be considered a contributing factor to a decrease in myocardial ischemic injury. In both experiments 1 and 2 no significant change in left atrial pressure was found after diltiazem. In the present study, contractility of the ischemic myocardium was not measured. But if diltiazem depresses contractility of the ischemic myocardium selectively as does verapamil, a similar Ca^{2+} antagonist (16), myocardial ischemic injury can be depressed by reduction of not only heart rate but also contractility of the ischemic myocardium.

Myocardial Blood Flow

The use of tracer microsphere technique provides a means of repeatedly determining the distribution of blood flow to various regions of evolving myocardial infarcts and, hence, of assessing collateral flow. Changes of flow distribution in the acute infarcts of conscious dogs in the present study resembled those found by Schaper and Pasyk (13). However, flow measurements by the tracer microsphere technique in the necrotic myocardium are reported to be in error because of microsphere loss, as evidenced by Jugdutt and Becker (2). Therefore, in the present study, only changes in flow after saline or diltiazem were considered for discussion. In the present investigation, a continuous infusion of diltiazem from 15 min to 24 hr after LAD occlusion increased myocardial blood flow significantly in the subepicardial layer of the ischemic area. This increase in flow may suggest a beneficial effect of diltiazem in salvaging ischemic myocardium instead of producing transmural necrosis because diltiazem did not increase factors contributing to myocardial oxygen demand such as heart rate, blood pressure, and left atrial pressure.

Schaper (12) and Schaper and Pasyk (13) demonstrated that an increase in collateral flow was found to start in the subepicardial layer of dogs 4 to 6 hr after coronary occlusion and, by microscopic examination of the collaterals, that these vessels, which were surrounded by hypoxic myocardium, were maximally dilated from the moment of acute coronary occlusion. An increase in collateral flow is considered to be very difficult to achieve owing to the high resistance of the collaterals after acute coronary occlusion (12,13). However, the present study demonstrated that, although intravenous administration of diltiazem for 20 sec did not increase flow in the ischemic myocardium 30 min after acute LAD occlusion [experiment 1(a)], continuous infusion of the drug increased flow in the ischemic myocardium 24 hr after coronary occlusion (experiment 2). The subepicardial location of interarterial anastomoses in the dog heart may account for the significantly greater increase of flow after diltiazem in the subepicardium than in the subendocardium.

The mechanism by which a continuous infusion of diltiazem did not increase flow significantly in the nonischemic area and yet increased flow significantly in the ischemic subepicardial layer remains unknown. The following mechanism is considered. Diltiazem would dilate the collateral vessels located in the subepicardial layers within 24 hr after acute coronary occlusion. According to the results obtained by Takeda et al. (18) on the isolated perfused dog heart supported by a donor, diltiazem produced a decrease in the large vessel resistance as well as in the total resistance, although reduction of the large vessel resistance lasted a little longer. The ischemic area is dependent on collateral circulation for maintenance of viability, and dilatation of the large coronary arteries as well as of the collaterals by diltiazem may cause an increase in the distal pressure in the occluded LAD and, thus, may increase blood flow to the ischemic area via dilated collateral vessels. An increase of flow in the ischemic area may be distributed predominantly to the subepicardial layer as compared with the subendocardium because the no-reflow phenomenon is observed to be greater in the subendocardium as compared with the subepicardium.

Furthermore, in contrast to nitroglycerin, diltiazem did not reduce left atrial pressure and preload of the left ventricle. The latter (no reduction of preload) may explain why there was no increase in subendocardial flow and subendocardial/subepicardial flow ratio. In the nonischemic area, diltiazem tended to increase flow, especially in the subepicardial layer, but this increase was not significant, probably because the resistance of the coronary arterioles, which is the main control of the flow in the nonischemic myocardium, was not affected significantly by diltiazem under the experimental conditions. A decrease in the frequency of premature ventricular contraction after diltiazem could also be considered as one of the mechanisms by which flow in the ischemic area was increased. Further study is required to determine if the increase in subepicardial flow by diltiazem is too slow in onset to be a great value in the prevention of transmural ischemic necrosis. A short period of injection of diltiazem in chronic myocardial infarction increased myocardial blood flow in the ischemic area as well as in the nonischemic myocardium, probably because of dilatation of the well-developed collaterals as well as of the resistive coronary arteries.

These results suggest that a part of the acutely ischemic subepicardium may be saved, that irreversibility of ischemia may be delayed, and that collateral flow to the ischemic area in acute and chronic myocardial infarction may be increased by diltiazem.

Infarct Size Estimated by Serum CPK

In experiment 2, the relationship between the infarct size estimated by the method of Shell et al. (14) and the size of the ischemic area estimated by flow measurement was poor. These findings coincided with the results obtained by Roe (10). It was impossible to distinguish a small from a moderately large infarct estimated as an area with flow less than 30% of the control nonischemic area 24 hr after LAD occlusion. Further studies on histological determination of infarct size in these animals are underway and will be reported in the furture.

Other Aspects of the Use of Diltiazem

Further analysis is required to determine if a significant decrease in premature ventricular contraction by diltiazem 22 to 24 hr after LAD occlusion resulted from an increase of flow in the ischemic subepicardium. Further studies are required to know if diltiazem can diminish histopathological infarct size and improve myocardial function in the acutely ischemic myocardium without significant side effects. Unfortunately, its use may be limited by the following side effect. Diltiazem, a coronary vasodilater, antagonizes Ca^{2+} and causes a reduction in the contraction of cardiac ventricle and vascular smooth muscles (7,8). It has a mild negative inotropic effect (11) and has been reported to exacerbate atrioventricular block and precipitate cardiac decompensation, a frequent complication of acute myocardial infarction (3). In the present study, however, continuous infusion did not cause an elevation of mean left atrial pressure, second degree atrioventricular block, or a decrease of arterial pressure in the acute myocardial infarction, which suggests that the potential undesirable effects mentioned above were avoided.

SUMMARY

The intravenous administration of 100 μg/kg of diltiazem over 20 sec reduced significantly the average ST segment elevation in dogs with acute coronary ligation without increasing flow in the ischemic myocardium. The continuous infusion of diltiazem for 24 hr, beginning 15 min after coronary occlusion, caused a significant increase of subepicardial flow in the ischemic myocardium 24 hr following occlusion and a significant reduction of the frequency of premature ventricular contraction 22 and 24 hr after occlusion. The administration of diltiazem increased myocardial flow of both ischemic and nonischemic areas in dogs infarcted about 3 weeks previously.

ACKNOWLEDGMENTS

The study was supported in part by grants from the Education Ministry of Japan (344044). The authors thank Miss Y. Tanaka, R. Hatao, and R. Kawashima for their assistance.

REFERENCES

1. Braunwald, E., and Maroko, P. (1974): The reduction of infarct size—an idea whose time (for testing) has come. *Circulation,* 50:206–209.
2. Jugdutt, B., and Becker, L. (1977): Microsphere loss from necrotic myocardium after experimental coronary artery occlusion. *Circulation (Suppl. III),* 56:III-90(Abstract).
3. Koseisho-Yakumukyoku (Ministry of Health and Welfare of Japan) Nihon-Ijishinpoh (1978): May 6:108–109 (in Japanese).
4. Maroko, P., and Braunwald, E. (1976): Effects of metabolic and pharmacologic interventions on myocardial infarct size following coronary occlusion. *Circulation (Suppl. I),* 53:I-162–I-168.
5. Maroko, P., Kjekshus, J. K., Sobel, B. E., Watanabe, T., Covell, J. W., Ross, J., Jr., and Braunwald, E. (1971): Factors influencing infarct size following experimental coronary artery occlusion. *Circulation,* 43:67–82.
6. Nagao, T., Murata, S., and Sato, M. (1975): Effects of diltiazem (CRD-401) on developed coronary collaterals in the dog. *Jpn. J. Pharmacol.,* 25:281–288.
7. Nakajima, H., Hoshiyama, M., Yamashita, K., and Kiyomoto, A. (1975): Effect of diltiazem on electrical and mechanical activity of isolated cardiac ventricular muscle of guinea pig. *Jpn. J. Pharmacol.,* 25:383–392.
8. Nakajima, H., Nosaka, K., and Hoshiyama, M. (1977): Effects of diltiazem on the positive and vasoconstrictor responses to ouabain *in vitro. Jpn. J. Pharmacol.,* 27:910–914.
9. Nakamura, M., Matsuguchi, H., Mitsutake, A., Kikuchi, Y., Takeshita, A., Nakagaki, O., and Kuroiwa, A. (1977): The effect of graded coronary stenosis on myocardial blood flow and left ventricular wall motion. *Basic Res. Cardiol.,* 72:479–491.
10. Roe, C. R. (1977): Validity of estimating myocardial infarct size from serial measurements of enzyme activity in the serum. *Clin. Chem.,* 23:1807–1812.
11. Sato, M., Nagao, T., Yamaguchi, I., Nakajima, H., and Kiyomoto, A. (1971): Pharmacological studies on a new 1.5-Benzothiazepine derivative (CRD-401). *Arzneim-Forsch.,* 21:1338–1343.
12. Schaper, W. (1971): *The Collateral Circulation of the Heart.* North-Holland, Amsterdam.
13. Schaper, W., and Pasyk, S. (1976): Influence of collateral flow on the ischemic tolerance of the heart following acute and subacute coronary occlusion. *Circulation (Suppl. I),* 53:I-57–I-62.
14. Shell, W. E., Lavelle, J. F., Covell, J. W., and Sobel, B. E. (1973): Early estimation of myocardial damage in conscious dogs and patients with evolving acute myocardial infarction. *J. Clin. Invest.,* 52:2579–2590.
15. Singh, B. N., Smith, H. J., and Norris, R. M. (1975): Reduction in infarct size following experimental coronary occlusion by administration of verapamil. In: *Recent Advances in Studies on Cardiac Structure and Metabolism. Volume 10. The Metabolism of Contraction,* edited by P. E. Roy and G. Rona, pp. 435–452. University Park Press, Baltimore.
16. Smith, H. J., Goldstein, R. A., Griffith, J. M., Kent, K. M., and Epstein, St. E. (1976): Regional

contractility—selective depression of ischemic myocardium by verapamil. *Circulation,* 54:629–635.

17. Smith, H. S., Singh, B. N., Nisbet, H. D., and Norris, R. M. (1975): Effects of verapamil on infarct size following experimental coronary artery occlusion. *Cardiovasc. Res.,* 9:569–578.
18. Takeda, K., Nakagawa, Y., Katano, Y., and Imai, S. (1977): Effects of coronary vasodilators on large and small coronary arteries of dogs. *Jpn. Heart J.,* 18:92–101.
19. Yasue, H., Omote, S., Takizawa, A., Nagao, M., Miwa, K., Kato, H., Tanaka, S., and Akiyama, F. (1978): Pathogenesis and treatment of angina pectoris at rest as seen from its response to various drugs. *Jpn. Circ. J.,* 42:1–10.

Ischemic Myocardium and Antianginal Drugs,
edited by M. M. Winbury and Y. Abiko.
Raven Press, New York © 1979.

Protection of Ischemic Myocardium by Treatment with Nifedipine

Philip D. Henry and Richard E. Clark

Cardiovascular Division, Department of Internal Medicine, Barnes Hospital, Washington University School of Medicine, St. Louis, Missouri 63110

Current evidence supports the concept that intracellular accumulation of Ca^{2+} plays an important role in mediating ischemic myocardial injury. Myocardial reperfusion after temporary ischemia (16) or perfusion with Ca^{2+}-free perfusate (10) has been reported to result in accumulations of intracellular Ca^{2+} and in explosive deteriorations in myocardial structure and function. Deposits of Ca^{2+} have also been described in the cardiac lesions produced by the administration of large amounts of catecholamines (5) and in the cardiomyopathy of the Syrian hamster (11).

Recently, Fleckenstein (6) and collaborators have delineated a group of compounds referred to as Ca^{2+} antagonists, which inhibit the contractile activity of cardiac and smooth muscle by blocking the inward movement of Ca^{2+} into cells. Fleckenstein (5) further demonstrated that pretreatment with the Ca^{2+} antagonists verapamil and D600 protected rats against catecholamine-induced cardiac necrosis and Ca^{2+} accumulation. As myocardial ischemia results in the release of catecholamines from the heart (15) and as there are some similarities between the cardiac lesions produced by ischemia and catecholamines (1), we wondered if Ca^{2+} antagonists might exert a protective effect on ischemic cardiac muscle. In a previous study (8), we have shown that nifedipine increases collateral perfusion of the ischemic myocardium and decreases ischemic injury in conscious dogs subjected to coronary occlusion.

In the present experiments, we have examined the effects of nifedipine on the globally ischemic heart *in vitro* and *in vivo*. Results demonstrate that this Ca^{2+} antagonist prevents ischemic myocardial contracture and the accumulation of intracellular Ca^{2+} and markedly improves the functional recovery of the heart after hypo- or normothermic cardiopulmonary bypass.

MATERIALS AND METHODS

Isolated Perfused Heart Preparation

Rabbit hearts were isolated and perfused retrograde at 37°C through the aorta as previously described (9). The perfusate contained (mM): NaCl, 118;

KCl, 3.8; KH_2PO_4, 1.2; $CaCl_2$, 1.5; $MgSO_4$, 1.2; $NaHCO_3$, 25; and glucose, 5. After equilibration with a 5% CO_2–95% O_2 gas mixture, the pH was approximately 7.4. The rate of perfusion was maintained at 22 ml/min with a roller pump. A latex balloon mounted around a micromanometer (Konigsberg model P3.5) was inserted into the left ventricular cavity for measurement of left ventricular pressure and its first-time derivative, dP/dt. These measurements were recorded with Brush amplifiers and a Brush recorder. The balloon was filled slowly with deaerated saline with the use of a micrometer syringe until end-diastolic pressure stabilized between 5 and 8 mm Hg. A bipolar electrode was attached to the right ventricular free wall, and the heart was paced at 180/min with rectangular impulses (1 msec; voltage 10% above threshold) provided by a Grass stimulator. Thus, in this preparation, major determinants of cardiac performance, including ventricular preload and afterload, cardiac frequency, coronary flow, perfusate composition, and temperature, were controlled. All hearts were equilibrated for 30 min at a flow rate of 22 ml/min. Then slow perfusion (0.2 ml/min; ~ 5 ml/100 g fresh myocardium/min) with perfusate containing nifedipine or its vehicle was started and maintained for 60 min. The drug, or its vehicle in control experiments, was infused with a syringe pump into the perfusion system at a rate not exceeding 1% of the total flow. The concentration of the drug reaching the heart was calculated on the basis of its concentration in the syringe and the flow rates of the two pumps. To protect the light-sensitive nifedipine, the whole infusion system was covered with opaque materials. In some experiments, high flow (22 ml/min) without nifedipine was reinstituted (reperfusion) at the end of the slow flow interval. In other experiments, hearts at the end of perfusion were used to determine the ventricular wet weight/dry weight ratio. The large vessels and atria were removed and the ventricles were opened, blotted, weighed, and subsequently taken to a constant dry weight in an oven at 80°C.

Biochemical Procedures

We utilized the Ca^{2+} content of the mitochondrial fraction as an index of cell Ca^{2+}, using copper as a mitochondrial marker. This approach is based on the findings that most of the Ca^{2+} accumulating in ischemic myocardium is recovered in the mitochondrial fraction and that copper in blood-free myocardium is an index of mitochondria and mitochondrial cristae (9). It is assumed that accumulation of mitochondrial Ca^{2+} is a reflection of an increased Ca^{2+} in the myoplasm, since a rise in extramitochondrial Ca^{2+} is the major factor determining energy-linked Ca^{2+} uptake by mitochondria (9). At the end of the perfusions (or, in control experiments, immediately after quick removal of the heart from the chest of the animal), hearts were immersed in ice-cold isolation medium containing mannitol (210 mM), sucrose (70 mM), and Tris-HCl (pH 7.4; 10 mM), and simultaneously perfused retrograde with 200 ml of the same medium. If not otherwise specified, ruthenium red, (500 μM) was added to preparative solutions to inhibit Ca^{2+} uptake by mitochondria during cell fractionation (9). In some experiments, nifedipine (10^{-7} M), was included also. The myocardium was homogenized, and the mitochondrial fraction was isolated as previously described (9). Ca^{2+} and copper in whole homogenates and mitochondrial fractions were measured by atomic absorption spectrophotometry in a Perkin-Elmer apparatus (model 303) (9).

Cardiopulmonary Bypass in Dogs

For studies of global myocardial ischemia, dogs were subjected to cardiopulmonary bypass as previously described (3). In one series of experiments, conditions were designed to mimic those currently utilized clinically and included systemic hypothermia (28°C), topical hypothermia, and priming with Ringer's lactate containing glucose (30 mM), KCl (40 mM), insulin (60 U/liter), and mannitol (60 mM). After institution of hypothermia, the animals were placed on total cardiopulmonary bypass for 2 hr. A systemic loading dose of nifedipine (20 μg/kg) was administered, followed by continuous infusion of nifedipine and saline into the aortic root at a rate of 5 μg/kg/hr. The amount of saline infused into the aorta (2.5 ml/kg/hr) was the same for treated and control animals. No drug was administered before or after bypass.

In other experiments, dogs were subjected to 1 hr of cardiopulmonary bypass under normothermic conditions (37°C). In these experiments, nifedipine in saline was administered into the aortic root at the rate of 2 μg/kg/hr. The amount of saline infused into the aorta was 12 ml/kg/hr in both control and treated animals. Additional control experiments were performed in which Normosol or saline containing 25 mM KCl or a cardioplegic solution was infused at the same rate of 12 ml/kg/hr. The cardioplegic solution contained (mM): Na, 154; K, 24.3; Mg, 2.7; Cl, 115; HCO_3, 23; acetate, 23; and gluconate, 22. The solution also contained 60 mM glucose, insulin (1.8 U/liter), and lidocaine (0.4 g/liter).

RESULTS

Isolated Heart Experiments

A representative record of an isovolumic left heart preparation subjected to 60 min of low flow (0.2 ml/min) is illustrated in Fig. 1 (top). Throughout the experiment, the heart was paced at a frequency of 180/min. Note that once ischemic standstill has occurred, the ventricle undergoes progressive ischemic contracture. Ventricular pressure at the end of the ischemic period exceeds 50 mm Hg. With subsequent reperfusion, end-diastolic pressure remains markedly elevated, which indicates persistent myocardial stiffness. In addition, the heart is arrhythmic despite ventricular pacing. Figure 1 (bottom) shows the response of a heart subjected to exactly the same protocol except that nifedipine (10^{-7} M) was added to the perfusate during (but not before or after) low flow.

CONTROL

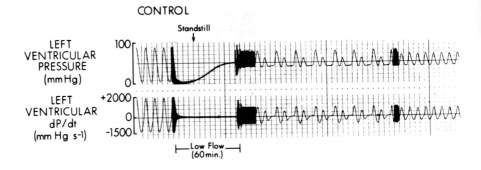

NIFEDIPINE

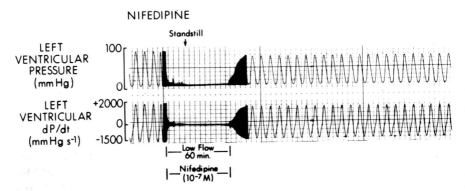

FIG. 1. Inhibition of ischemic ventricular contracture by nifedipine. Perfusion experiments with paced isovolumic left heart preparations were performed as described in "Methods." Standstill refers to no visible ventricular activity and no pulsatile pressure on tracings recorded with a second recorder at a paper speed of 25 mm/sec and a full scale of 100 mm Hg. Low flow refers to a rate of perfusion of 0.2 ml/min. Fast and slow (black areas) segments of the tracings were recorded at a paper speed of 25 mm/sec and 1 mm/min, respectively.

As in the control experiment, there is a precipitous decline in cardiac contractility followed by ventricular standstill. However, in sharp contrast to the control experiments, no contracture develops. Furthermore, with reperfusion, end-diastolic pressure remains low, and there is a striking recovery in developed pressure and dP/dt. Results of the experiments depicted in Fig. 1 are diagrammatically summarized in Figs. 2 and 3.

Results of measurements of calcium, copper, and protein in perfused hearts and in hearts processed immediately after sacrifice of the animal are summarized in Table 1. Note that with the protocol used in this study, inclusion of nifedipine or ruthenium red in the preparative solution did not appreciably influence the Ca^{2+} content in the mitochondrial fraction. Furthermore, perfusion at high flow resulted only in a minor increase in mitochondrial Ca^{2+}. On the other hand, 60 min of low flow without nifedipine increased the Ca^{2+} value more

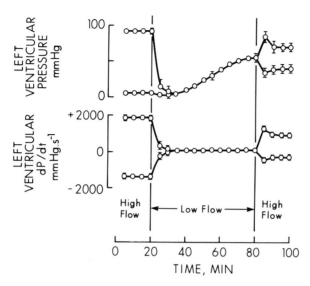

FIG. 2. Ischemic contracture in isovolumic left heart preparations ($n = 8$). Perfusions were performed as described in "Methods" and illustrated in Fig. 1 *(top)*. High and low flow refer to a flow of 22 and 0.2 ml/min, respectively. Buffer during low flow contained < 0.1% of the vehicle of nifedipine (final ethanol and polyethylene glycol concentrations both less than 0.015%). Data points indicate mean ± SE.

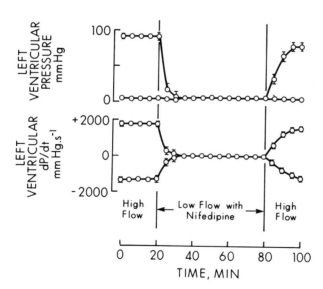

FIG. 3. Inhibition of ischemic contracture by 10^{-7} M nifedipine ($n = 8$). Experiments were performed exactly as described in "Methods" and illustrated in Fig. 1 except that the vehicle contained nifedipine to yield a final drug concentration of 10^{-7} M. No nifedipine was administered before or after the period of low flow. Data points indicate mean ± SE.

TABLE 1. *Calcium and copper in mitochondrial fraction*[a]

	Calcium ng atom mg protein	Copper ng atom mg protein	Calcium/Copper	Copper in mitochondrial fraction (%)	Protein in mitochondrial fraction (%)
No perfusion[b] −N (8)	6.2 ± 0.3	1.37 ± 0.05	4.53 ± 0.23	10.9 ± 0.4	4.01 ± 0.22
+N (8)	6.3 ± 0.3	1.36 ± 0.06	4.63 ± 0.24	11.4 ± 0.5	4.12 ± 0.23
−R (7)	6.8 ± 0.4	1.38 ± 0.04	4.93 ± 0.29	10.7 ± 0.4	4.10 ± 0.19
60 min −N (7)	7.6 ± 0.4	1.38 ± 0.06	5.51 ± 0.41	11.6 ± 0.5	4.21 ± 0.25
high flow[c] +N (8)	7.4 ± 0.4	1.34 ± 0.06	5.52 ± 0.43	12.0 ± 0.7	4.05 ± 0.28
60 min −N (10)	28.2 ± 1.9	1.41 ± 0.05	19.9 ± 1.61	9.2 ± 0.9	3.41 ± 0.21
low flow[d] +N (10)	8.0 ± 0.5	1.30 ± 0.07	6.15 ± 0.55	10.8 ± 0.7	4.15 ± 0.27
60 min low −N (11)	55.5 ± 4.8	1.29 ± 0.09	42.65 ± 3.9	6.8 ± 0.7	2.52 ± 0.21
flow + 10 min +N (12)	10.0 ± 0.6	1.33 ± 0.10	7.52 ± 0.63	9.4 ± 0.7	3.50 ± 0.24
reperfusion[e] −R (9)	58.6 ± 6.0	1.31 ± 0.12	44.73 ± 4.8	6.2 ± 0.8	2.31 ± 0.30

[a] Percentages of copper or protein in the mitochondrial fraction are expressed as percentages of the total myocardial copper or protein in the whole homogenate. Values are means ± SE.

[b] No perfusion: Hearts processed immediately after sacrifice of the animal without Langendorff perfusion; in these preparations, −N and +N refer to the absence or presence, respectively, of 10^{-7} M nifedipine in the preparative solutions, and −R indicates that ruthenium red was omitted from all preparative solutions. Numbers in parentheses indicate the number of hearts studied.

[c] High flow: Perfusion at 22 ml/min; in perfused hearts, −N and +N refer to the addition of vehicle alone or vehicle + nifedipine (10^{-7} M), respectively, to the perfusate during the experimental perfusion period (60 min). Numbers in parentheses indicate the number of hearts studied.

[d] Low flow: Perfusion at 0.2 ml/min; −N and +N as in high flow. Numbers in parentheses indicate the number of hearts studied.

[e] Reperfusion: −R indicates that perfusion was carried out without nifedipine and that ruthenium red was omitted from all preparative solutions; −N and +N, as in high flow and low flow. The numbers in parentheses indicate the numbers of hearts studied.

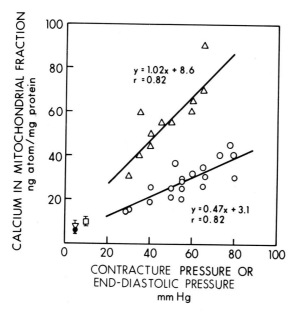

FIG. 4. Relationship between ischemic contracture and accumulation of calcium in the mitochondrial fraction. Perfusions were performed as described in "Methods." Mitochondrial fractions were prepared with solutions containing ruthenium red. *Solid circle with bars,* After a standard equilibration period, hearts were perfused at 22 ml/min for 60 min with buffer containing no nifedipine ($n = 7$). *Open inverted triangle with bars,* Perfusions at low flow (0.2 ml/min) for 60 min with buffer containing nifedipine (10^{-7} M) and its vehicle ($n = 9$). *Open square with bars,* After a 60-min-period of low flow with nifedipine, hearts were reperfused at 22 ml/min for 10 min with buffer containing no nifedipine ($n = 10$). *Open circles,* 60-min perfusions at low flow with buffer containing vehicle without nifedipine. *Open triangles,* 60 min of low flow with buffer containing vehicle without nifedipine, followed by 10 min of reperfusion. Data points represent means ± SE and are from the same experiments as those summarized in Figs. 2 and 3 and Table 2.

than fourfold, and subsequent reperfusion for 10 min produced a further marked increase. In contrast, in nifedipine-treated hearts subjected to low flow with or without reperfusion, accumulation of Ca^{2+} in the mitochondrial fraction remained modest.

Figure 4 shows the relationship between myocardial stiffness, as reflected by the nonpulsatile ventricular pressure at the end of the low-flow period (contracture pressure) or by the end-diastolic pressure after 10 min of reperfusion, and accumulation of Ca^{2+} in the mitochondrial fraction. It can be seen that increasing myocardial stiffness was associated with increasing Ca^{2+} values. In addition, the diagram shows that reperfusion enhanced the accumulation of Ca^{2+}. Treatment with nifedipine prevented ischemic myocardial stiffness as well as accumulation of Ca^{2+}.

TABLE 2. Hemodynamics after 2 hr of hypothermic bypass with and without nifedipine

Determination[a]	Control dogs (n = 7)			Drug-treated dogs (n = 6)		
	Before	After	p Value[b]	Before	After	p Value[b]
LAP (mm Hg)	3.5	9.3	< 0.001	5.7	10	< 0.001
HR (beats/min)	157	155	NS	159	150	NS
LVP_{max} (mm Hg)	156	87	< 0.001	142	140	NS
LVEDP (mm Hg)	0.3	14	< 0.001	1.0	7.7	< 0.001
CVP (mm Hg)	4.9	9.6	< 0.001	4.9	7.3	NS
MAP (mm Hg)	115	63.7	< 0.001	81	90	NS
CO (liters/min)	2,300	700	< 0.001	1,820	1,320	< 0.003
SV (ml/beat)	14.6	4.52	< 0.001	11.5	8.8	NS
LV dP/dt (mm Hg/sec)	3,981	1,853	< 0.001	3,406	2,766	< 0.05

[a]LAP, left atrial pressure; HR, heart rate; LVP_{max}, peak left ventricular pressure; LVEDP, left ventricular end-diastolic pressure; CVP, central venous pressure; MAP, mean arterial pressure; CO, cardiac output; SV, stroke volume; LV dP/dt, maximum rate of rise of left ventricular pressure.
[b]NS, not significant.

TABLE 3. *Hemodynamics after 1 hr of normothermic bypass with and without pharmacological intervention*

| | | 1 hr on bypass at 37°C plus 2 hr off bypass | | | | |
| | | Control groups | | | Treatment groups | |
Determination[a]	Prebypass	Normal saline	Normal saline + 25 meq/liter KCl	Normosol-R pH 7.4	Clinical cardioplegic solution	Nifedipine in saline
Stroke work index (g-m/m²)	22.4 ± 1.0	7.1 ± 0.6	11.4 ± 1.7	10.6 ± 0.5	16.9 ± 2.9	21.7 ± 5.8
% Change from preischemic value	—	−68	−49	−53	−25	−3
LV dP/dt (mm Hg/sec)	3500 ± 188	2525 ± 340	2350 ± 210	2300 ± 264	2566 ± 550	3290 ± 452
% Change from preischemic value	—	−28	−33	−34	−27	−6
LVEDP (mm Hg)	8.3 ± 0.9	18.3 ± 2.9	17.8 ± 3.3	15.3 ± 5.5	15.7 ± 0.9	11.4 ± 2.8
% Change from preischemic value	—	+120	+113	+84	+88	+37
Number of dogs	21	4	4	3	3	5

[a] Abbreviations as in Table 2.

Cardiopulmonary Bypass Experiments

Table 2 summarizes hemodynamic data of control and nifedipine-treated dogs after 2 hr of hypothermic cardiopulmonary bypass. Control animals exhibited very severe depression of cardiac performance, and attempts to wean the dogs from the bypass with various supportive maneuvers (variation in preload, norepinephrine, $CaCl_2$, or ouabain) were unsuccessful. In contrast, dogs treated with nifedipine showed a remarkable preservation of cardiac function, compatible with survival.

The protective effects on the globally ischemic heart were also evident in dogs subjected to 1 hr of normothermic cardiopulmonary bypass. Hemodynamic measurements 2 hr after bypass for animals treated with nifedipine and other regimens are summarized in Table 3. As in the hypothermic bypass experiments, nifedipine-treated animals exhibited a remarkable preservation of cardiac function compared to the control dogs.

DISCUSSION

Results of the present study demonstrate that isolated hearts perfused at low flow undergo a progressive contracture that is associated with an accumulation of Ca^{2+} in the mitochondrial cell fraction prepared from ventricular myocardium. In addition, nifedipine, a dihydropyridine derivative that antagonizes the effects of Ca^{2+} on cardiac and smooth muscle (2,7,12,13), prevents myocardial contracture and accumulation of Ca^{2+} and improves mechanical recovery after reperfusion. The salient finding of the perfused heart experiments is the striking correlation between cardiomechanical changes typical of ischemia and the accumulation of Ca^{2+} in the mitochondrial fraction.

Incomplete or delayed myocardial relaxation and decreased myocardial compliance during episodes of myocardial ischemia have been demonstrated in patients suffering from coronary artery disease (14) and in patients undergoing cardiopulmonary bypass (4). The observation that nifedipine inhibits ischemic contracture in the globally ischemic heart *in vitro* suggested to us that this drug may be potentially useful for the preservation of the ischemic heart *in vivo*. The remarkable preservation of cardiac function in nifedipine-treated dogs undergoing cardiopulmonary bypass observed in this study is consistent with this assumption.

In conclusion, the present experiments demonstrate that nifedipine exerts striking protective effects on the globally ischemic heart *in vitro* and *in vivo*. Results suggest that nifedipine may provide a new tool for the pharmacological protection of the globally ischemic heart in the clinical setting.

REFERENCES

1. Baroldi, G. (1975): Different types of myocardial necrosis in coronary heart disease: A pathophysiologic review of their functional significance. *Am. Heart J.,* 89:742–752.

2. Bayer, R., Rodenkirchen, R., Kaufmann, R., Lee, J. H., and Hennekes, R. (1977): The effects of nifedipine on contraction and monophasic action potential of isolated cat myocardium. *Naunyn Schmiedebergs Arch. Pharmacol.,* 301:29–37.

3. Clark, R. E., Ferguson, T. C., West, P. N., Shuchleib, R. C., and Henry, P. D. (1977): Pharmacological preservation of the ischemic heart. *Ann. Thorac. Surg.,* 24:307–314.

4. Cooley, D. A., Reul, G. J., and Wukasch, D. C. (1972): Ischemic contracture of the heart: "Stone heart." *Am. J. Cardiol.,* 29:575–583.

5. Fleckenstein, A. (1970): Die Zügelung des Myocardstoffwechsels durch Verapamil. *Arzneim. Forsch.,* 20:1317–1322.

6. Fleckenstein, A. (1975): Fundamentale Herz und Gefässwirkungen Ca⁺⁺-antagonistischer Koronartherapeutika. *Med. Klin.,* 70:1665–1674.

7. Grün, G., and Fleckenstein, A. (1972): Die elektromechanische Entkoppelung der glatten Gefässmuskulatur als Grundprinzip der Coronardilatation durch 4-(2'-Nitrophenyl-)-2-6-dimethyl-1,4-dihydropyridine-3,5-dicarbonsäure-dimethylester (BAY a 1040, Nifedipine). *Arzneim. Forsch.* 22:334–344.

8. Henry, P. D., Shuchleib, R., Borda, L. J., Roberts, R., Williamson, J. R., and Sobel, B. E. (1978): Effects of nifedipine on myocardial perfusion and ischemic injury in dogs. *Circ. Res.,* 43:372–380.

9. Henry, P. D., Shuchleib, R., Davis, J., Weiss, E. S., and Sobel, B. E. (1977): Myocardial contracture and accumulation of mitochondrial calcium in ischemic rabbit heart. *Am. J. Physiol.,* 233:H677–H684.

10. Holland, C. E., and Olson, R. E. (1975): Prevention by hypothermia of paradoxical calcium necrosis in cardiac muscle. *J. Mol. Cell. Cardiol.,* 7:917–928.

11. Jasmin, J., and Proschek, L. (1979): Prevention of myocardial degeneration in hamsters with hereditary cardiomyopathy. *Excerpta Medica (in press).*

12. Kaufmann, R. (1977): Differenzierung verschiedener Kalzium-Antagonisten. *Muench. Med. Wochenschr.,* 119:6–11.

13. Kohlhardt, M., and Fleckenstein, A. (1977): Inhibition of the slow inward current by nifedipine in mammalian myocardium. *Naunyn Schmiedebergs Arch. Pharmacol.,* 298:267–272.

14. McLaurin, L. P., Rolett, E. L., and Grossmann, W. (1973): Impaired left ventricular relaxation during pacing-induced ischemia. *Am. J. Cardiol.,* 32:751–757.

15. Shahab, L., Wollenberger, A., Haase, M., and Schiller, V. (1969): Noradrenalin-abgabe aus dem Hundherzen nach vorübergehender Okklusion einer Koronararterie *Acta Biol. Med. Ger.,* 22:135–143.

16. Shen, A. C., and Jennings, R. B. (1972): Myocardial calcium and magnesium in acute ischemic injury. *Am. J. Pathol.,* 67:417–440.

Ischemic Myocardium and Antianginal Drugs,
edited by M. M. Winbury and Y. Abiko.
Raven Press, New York © 1979.

Effects of Antianginal Drugs on Ischemic Myocardial Metabolism

Yasushi Abiko, Kazuo Ichihara, and Takashi Izumi

Department of Pharmacology, Asahikawa Medical College, Asahikawa 078-11, Japan

It is commonly accepted that antianginal drugs relieve an anginal attack by restoring myocardial oxygen balance which has been disturbed by either a decrease in oxygen supply or an increase in oxygen demand. An increase in coronary blood flow would result in an increase in oxygen supply to the heart, which would lead to a better oxygen balance providing that oxygen demand does not increase. Accordingly, considerable effort has been made to discover more potent coronary dilators that do not increase oxygen consumption of the heart. The results of clinical studies, however, do not support the view that coronary dilators that do not increase myocardial oxygen consumption are always effective antianginal drugs.

Our interest in the past 5 years has been to find a good index that reflects the state of the regional myocardial oxygen balance. If one could find a good index to the regional oxygen balance in the myocardium, one would be able to evaluate a drug for relieving an anginal attack or improving myocardial ischemia. It should be noted, however, that in a stricter sense one of the most important determinants of survival for living cells is not oxygen balance itself but energy balance (balance between energy production and utilization). Therefore, a fundamental approach to solving the problem of the mechanisms of action of antianginal drugs is to find a good index to myocardial energy balance.

Several methods have been developed for evaluating the myocardial oxygen or energy balance, e.g., efficiency of myocardial work (mechanical work/oxygen consumption), tissue oxygen tension (Po_2), $NAD^+/NADH$ ratio, redoximeter that reflects the amount of NADH in the tissue, etc. Every method, however, has weak points. We have tried to use metabolic changes as an index of myocardial oxygen or energy balance because myocardial metabolism shifts from aerobic to anaerobic immediately after hypoxia or ischemia. If cellular oxygenation is inadequate, anaerobic metabolism takes place; the tissue oxygen level decreases and the glycolytic intermediate levels increase, leading to a marked accumulation of lactate in the hypoxic or ischemic tissue. The levels of energy-rich phosphates decrease under these conditions, and the decrease in the levels of energy-rich phosphates reflects a disturbance of myocardial energy balance.

There is another problem in discussing the regional oxygen or energy balance in the myocardium. This relates to the difference in response to coronary artery occlusion between the endo- and epicardial layers. It has been recognized that the subendocardial layers become more ischemic than the subepicardial layers after coronary artery occlusion (18). This finding was supported by the studies using microspheres (4) and tissue oxygen electrodes (27). Therefore, a study on myocardial metabolic response to ischemia should be performed in both endo- and epicardial layers.

For these reasons we have studied, first, the effect of coronary artery ligation on the endo- and epicardial metabolism, and second, the effect of pretreatment with antianginal drugs on the metabolic response of the myocardium to coronary artery ligation.

METHODS

Technique in Animal Experiments

Mongrel dogs of either sex weighing about 11 kg were anesthetized with sodium pentobarbital (30 mg/kg, i.v.). Under artificial respiration, the left side of the thorax was opened to permit free access to the left ventricular wall. One of the small branches of the anterior descending coronary artery was dissected free from the adjacent tissues, and a silk thread was placed around the branch. The thread was used for ligating the coronary branch (coronary artery ligation) to produce a relatively small area of ischemia. Therefore, no serious arrhythmias occurred after coronary artery ligation. However, it was possible to observe the change in color of the ischemic myocardium. Drugs or vehicle (saline solution with or without 1% ethanol) were injected intravenously 5 or 10 min (usually 5 min) before coronary artery ligation. A single sample was

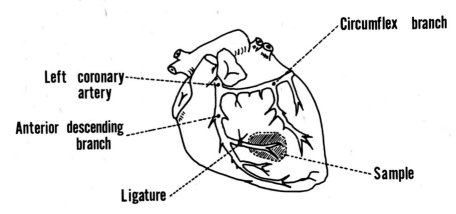

FIG. 1. Schematic illustration of ligature of a small branch of the anterior descending coronary artery and the region of the myocardium to be sampled.

taken from the ischemic region of individual dogs before and at various intervals after coronary ligation (Fig. 1). The sample before coronary artery ligation was defined as nonischemic and compared with the ischemic sample taken after coronary artery ligation. The myocardial sample was immediately pressed and frozen with freezing clamps (previously chilled with liquid nitrogen) so that the endo- and epicardial layers were on either side of the frozen sample. The time required to remove, press, and freeze the myocardial sample was less than 10 sec. The endo- and epicardial portions were then separated and cracked into fragments with a chisel (previously chilled with liquid nitrogen) and stored in liquid nitrogen.

Arterial blood pressure, heart rate, and electrocardiogram (limb lead II) were monitored until the myocardium was removed.

Analytical Technique

Each of the endo- and epicardial frozen fragments were divided into three samples.

Preparation of Samples

Sample 1

Each of the endo- and epicardial fragments was weighed (300 to 500 mg) and ground into a fine powder in a mortar chilled with liquid nitrogen. Special care was taken not to thaw the fragments in these procedures. The frozen tissue powder thus obtained was extracted with 5 volumes of 1 N $HClO_4$. The mixture containing tissue powder and perchloric acid was stirred for at least 3 min. The extract was centrifuged at $750 \times g$ for 10 min at 0°C, and the supernatant was gradually neutralized with KOH. This was recentrifuged at $750 \times g$ for 10 min, and the supernatant was used for determination of glucose-6-phosphate (G6P), lactate, adenosine triphosphate (ATP), and phosphocreatine (PCr).

Sample 2

Each of the endo- and epicardial frozen myocardial fragments was weighed (300 to 500 mg) and ground into powder. The frozen tissue powder was homogenized at −25°C in 10 volumes of 60% glycerol solution containing 20 mM KF and 1 mM EDTA ethylenediaminetetraacetic acid). The homogenate was centrifuged at $8,500 \times g$ for 10 min at −5°C. The supernatant was diluted fivefold in 0.1 M KF just before the determination of phosphorylase activity.

Sample 3

Each of the endo- and epicardial frozen fragments was weighed (100 to 150 mg) and analyzed for determination of tissue glycogen level.

Determination of Levels of Glycogen, G6P, Lactate, ATP, and PCr

The level of glycogen was measured by the method of Seifter et al. (24) and that of lactate by the method of Barker and Summerson (3). The levels of G6P, ATP, and PCr were measured enzymatically according to the method described by Bergmeyer (5).

Determination of Phosphorylase Activity

The phosphorylase activity was assayed by measuring inorganic phosphate (P_i) liberated by adding glucose-1-phosphate to the mixture that contained the supernatant of tissue sample 2 and the assay medium for phosphorylase described by Cornblath et al. (6). P_i was measured by the method of Fiske and Subbarow (8). The activity of phosphorylase a was assayed in the absence of 5'-adenosine monophosphate (5'-AMP), and that of total phosphorylase in the presence of 5'-AMP. Details of these procedures have been described (11).

Statistical Analysis

All values are expressed as mean $\pm$ SE, and a p value of 0.05 or less was considered significant (Student's t-test).

RESULTS AND DISCUSSION

Metabolic Response to Coronary Artery Ligation

The data shown in Figs. 2 to 7 consist of the results obtained in the nonischemic (before ligation) and the 1.5-, 3-, 7-, and 30-min ischemic groups. Each group consists of more than five dogs, usually six or seven dogs. There were seven series of experiments based on the drug that was injected before coronary artery ligation. Studies in which saline solution or saline solution containing 1% ethanol was injected were defined as control experiments. Saline solution containing 1% ethanol was used as a control for the nifedipine study because nifedipine was first dissolved in ethanol and then in saline solution.

Control Experiments

Figure 2 illustrates the metabolic response of the myocardium to coronary artery ligation (11). Saline solution was injected 5 min before coronary artery ligation in this series of experiments. The endo- and epicardial levels of glycogen, G6P, lactate, ATP, and PCr, and the activity of total phosphorylase and phosphorylase a are plotted against the time when the myocardial sample was taken. It should be noted that both endo- and epicardial samples were obtained from

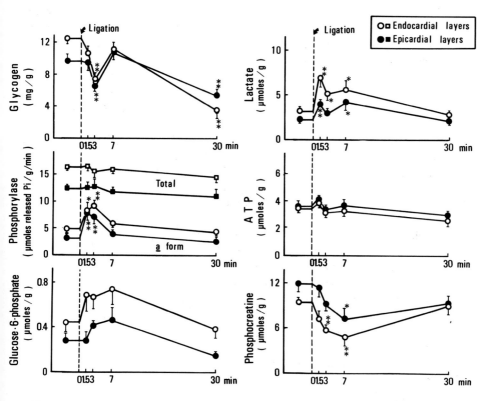

FIG. 2. Effect of coronary artery ligation on the endo- and epicardial levels of glycogen, glucose-6-phosphate, lactate, ATP, and phosphocreatine and on the activity of the total phosphorylase and phosphorylase a. The results obtained in the nonischemic and the 1.5-, 3-, 7-, and 30-min ischemic groups are indicated on the abscissa. Saline solution instead of drug solution was injected in this experiment. Each point represents mean ± SE. *, $p < 0.05$; **, $p < 0.01$ versus the level or activity in the nonischemic myocardium. (Data from Ichihara and Abiko, ref. 11.)

the same heart, but the myocardial samples in different groups were not taken from the same heart. In the nonischemic group, the endocardial glycogen level was significantly higher than the epicardial. This finding agrees with that of Jedeikin (16). It is of interest that the levels of G6P and lactate and the activities of total phosphorylase and phosphorylase a in the endocardial layers were also higher than those in the epicardial layers, whereas the level of PCr in the endocardial layers was lower than that in the epicardial, and the levels of ATP in both endo- and epicardial layers were similar.

Coronary artery ligation produced a transient decrease in the glycogen level, a transient increase in the activity of phosphorylase a, increases in the G6P and lactate levels, and a decrease in the PCr level. The level of ATP remained unchanged. The endocardial metabolic changes were more prominent than the epicardial changes. Since the transient decrease in the glycogen level was accompanied by a corresponding increase in the phosphorylase a activity, it is likely that the increase in the phosphorylase a activity is responsible for the rapid decrease in the glycogen level. Rapid increases in the G6P and lactate levels can be interpreted as a result of activation of phosphorylase and acceleration of glycogenolysis. It is likely that conversion of phosphorylase from b-form to a-form occurred immediately after coronary artery ligation because the activity of phosphorylase a increased without a change in the total phosphorylase activity. Conversion of phosphorylase from b-form to a-form can be produced by catecholamines, glucagon, and calcium ions. There is evidence that catecholamine release occurs in the myocardium exposed to hypoxia or ischemia (28). Therefore, catecholamines are probably responsible for the activation of phosphorylase after coronary artery ligation. An increase in the glycogen level was observed after the initial decrease during coronary artery ligation. This is probably due to an increase in glycogen synthesis and inhibition of glycogenolysis as a result of an increase in the G6P level (19,21). There is a question, however, as to why the lactate level does not continue to increase after coronary artery ligation. One possibility is that a rapid development of collateral vessels occurs by which lactate can be washed out, but there is no evidence showing such a rapid development of collateral vessels. Another possibility is that glycolytic flow (22) is inhibited after an initial acceleration (25) in the ischemic myocardium. The level of ATP did not change, but that of PCr decreased after coronary artery ligation. These findings suggest that all the mechanisms are functioning to maintain the intracellular ATP at a constant level because maintenance of the intracellular ATP level is essential for survival of living cells. However, if the ischemic area is more extensive and the duration of the ischemic period is more prolonged, the ATP level will decrease until irreversible damage is brought about.

Nitroglycerin Experiments

The metabolic response of the myocardium to coronary artery ligation in the presence of nitroglycerin is illustrated in Fig. 3 (13). Nitroglycerin (20 μg/ kg, i.v.) decreased systolic and diastolic blood pressures and increased heart rate. These changes were rapid but transient, and the blood pressure and heart rate returned to about 70 to 80% of the control values 5 min after the nitroglycerin injection, as demonstrated in our previous paper (2). The levels of metabolic intermediates of the myocardium in the nonischemic group of the nitroglycerin-pretreated dogs were not different from those of the saline-control dogs.

Coronary artery ligation was performed 5 min after the nitroglycerin injection. The glycogen level decreased slowly, but the phosphorylase a activity did not increase after coronary artery ligation. The latter was an unexpected result. The level of lactate increased, but the degree of the increase was not as marked as seen in the control experiments. The ATP and G6P levels in both layers

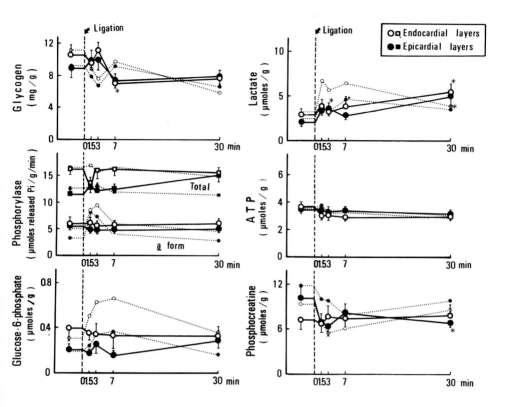

FIG. 3. Effect of pretreatment with nitroglycerin (20 μg/kg, i.v.) on the metabolic response to coronary artery ligation. *Solid lines,* results obtained in the presence of drug; *dotted lines,* results obtained in the absence of drug (saline control). Symbols are given in Fig. 2. (Data from Ichihara and Abiko, ref. 13.)

did not change after coronary ligation. The finding with respect to ATP level was just the same as seen in the control experiments. The epicardial PCr level decreased, but the endocardial PCr level did not change markedly after coronary artery ligation. These findings suggest that typical anaerobic metabolism does not occur after coronary artery ligation when the animals are pretreated with nitroglycerin. The reason for this is not clear at present. It is unlikely that a shift of myocardial metabolism from aerobic to anaerobic has been inhibited by the direct action of nitroglycerin on the myocardial metabolism because there is no clear evidence for the existence of direct inhibitory action of nitroglycerin on glycogenolysis and/or glycolysis. It is possible that nitroglycerin makes a shift of myocardial metabolism to anaerobic unnecessary, even after coronary artery ligation, because of an increase in perfusion of the ischemic area. Direct evidence that supports this assumption, however, is lacking. No matter what the mechanism is, treatment with nitroglycerin seems to be favorable for the prevention of ischemic changes of myocardium caused by coronary artery ligation.

Propranolol Experiments

The metabolic response of the myocardium to coronary artery ligation in the presence of propranolol is illustrated in Fig. 4 (14). Propranolol (1 mg/kg, i.v.) decreased heart rate from 158 ± 6 to 129 ± 4 beats/min but did not change blood pressure markedly.

In the nonischemic myocardium pretreated with propranolol, the levels of glycogen, ATP, and PCr were similar to those obtained in control experiments. However, phosphorylase activity and the levels of G6P and lactate were lower than in the control experiments.

As would be expected, coronary artery ligation did not increase the activity of phosphorylase a. It was also expected that the level of G6P would not change after coronary artery ligation in the presence of propranolol because glycogenoly-

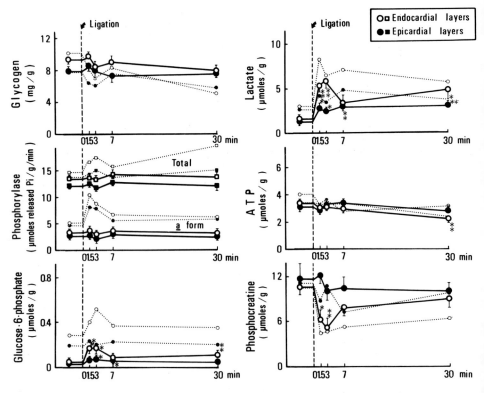

FIG. 4. Effect of pretreatment with propranolol (1 mg/kg, i.v.) on the metabolic response to coronary artery ligation. Symbols are given in Figs. 2 and 3. (Data from Ichihara and Abiko, ref. 14.)

sis would be inhibited by propranolol. However, a small and transient rise of G6P was noted after coronary artery ligation, especially in the endocardial layers. This is probably due to a supply of residual glucose from the ischemic extracellular space. The response of lactate to coronary artery ligation seems to be small compared with that seen in control experiments. This finding can be interpreted in terms of propranolol-induced inhibition of the acceleration of phosphorylase activity caused by coronary artery ligation. Thus propranolol inhibits glycogenolysis, and therefore the accumulation of glycolytic intermediates is inhibited even after coronary artery ligation. It should also be noted that the level of ATP did not change after coronary artery ligation and that the decrease in the PCr level caused by coronary artery ligation was smaller in the presence of propranolol than in the control experiments. Therefore, the pattern of metabolic changes after coronary artery ligation in the presence of propranolol is very similar to that obtained in the presence of nitroglycerin. Propranolol decreased heart rate, which led to less oxygen consumption of the heart. The action of propranolol on the heart rate is probably the reason why the levels of energy-rich phosphates do not decrease markedly, even after coronary artery ligation, while glycogenolysis is inhibited by propranolol.

Carteolol Experiments

Carteolol is one of the beta-adrenergic blocking agents (29). The metabolic response of the myocardium to coronary artery ligation in the presence of carteolol is illustrated in Fig. 5 (15). Carteolol (10 μg/kg, i.v.) was injected 5 min before coronary artery ligation. Heart rate decreased, but blood pressure remained unchanged after the carteolol injection.

The general pattern of metabolic response of the myocardium to coronary artery ligation in the presence of carteolol was similar to that obtained in the presence of propranolol. It is clear that the activity of phosphorylase a does not increase after coronary artery ligation in carteolol-pretreated dogs. From the results obtained in experiments with propranolol and carteolol, it is evident that beta-adrenergic receptors are involved in the increase in the activity of phosphorylase after coronary artery ligation.

Dipyridamole Experiments

Dipyridamole was chosen as one of the most potent coronary artery dilators. It has been proved that dipyridamole given intravenously (250 μg/kg) dilates the coronary vessels and increases coronary blood flow markedly (26). The metabolic response of the myocardium to coronary artery ligation in the presence of dipyridamole is illustrated in Fig. 6 (12). There was no marked difference between the saline-control and dipyridamole-pretreated dogs in the levels of glycolytic intermediates and energy-rich phosphates in the nonischemic myocardium.

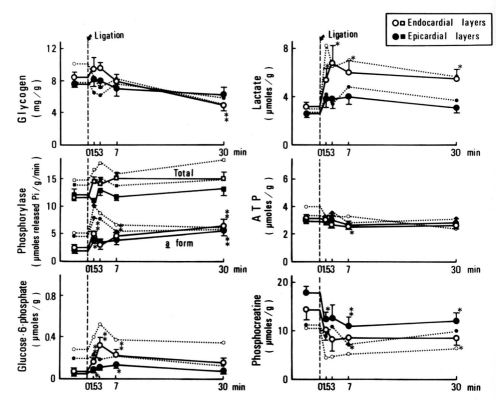

FIG. 5. Effect of pretreatment with carteolol (10 µg/kg, i.v.) on the metabolic response to coronary artery ligation. Symbols are given in Figs. 2 and 3. (Some data from Ichihara et al., ref. 15.)

After coronary artery ligation, the activity of phosphorylase and the levels of glycolytic intermediates increased. The pattern of changes in the levels of glycolytic intermediates in the dipyridamole-pretreated dogs was similar to that obtained in the saline-control dogs. These results suggest that dipyridamole does not influence markedly the metabolic response of the myocardium to coronary artery ligation.

Carbochromen Experiments

Chromonar (carbochromen) was also used as a potent coronary dilator. It has been reported that carbochromen increases the endocardial blood flow (9) and myocardial oxygen tension (17). The metabolic response of the myocardium to coronary artery ligation in the presence of carbochromen is illustrated in Fig. 7. Carbochromen (4 mg/kg, i.v.) was injected 10 min before coronary artery ligation. In nonischemic myocardium, it was noted that the activity of

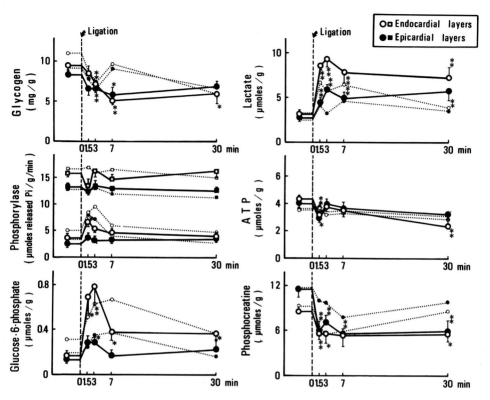

FIG. 6. Effect of pretreatment with dipyridamole (250 μg/kg, i.v.) on the metabolic response to coronary artery ligation. Symbols are given in Figs. 2 and 3. (Data from Ichihara and Abiko, ref. 12.)

phosphorylase a in both endo- and epicardial layers in carbochromen-pretreated dogs was higher than in the saline-control dogs. This evidence coincides with the result reported by Schraven et al. (23); carbochromen increases the tissue level of cyclic AMP.

After coronary artery ligation, the level of glycogen and the activity of phosphorylase decreased in dogs pretreated with carbochromen. The levels of G6P and lactate increased, and the level of PCr decreased after coronary artery ligation. The level of ATP, however, did not change even after coronary artery ligation. Thus the results obtained in carbochromen-pretreated dogs were similar to those obtained in saline-control dogs, except for the activity of phosphorylase in the nonischemic myocardium.

Calcium-Antagonist Experiments

It has been reported that, in the isolated perfused rat heart, increasing the concentration of calcium ions in the perfusion medium accelerates myocardial

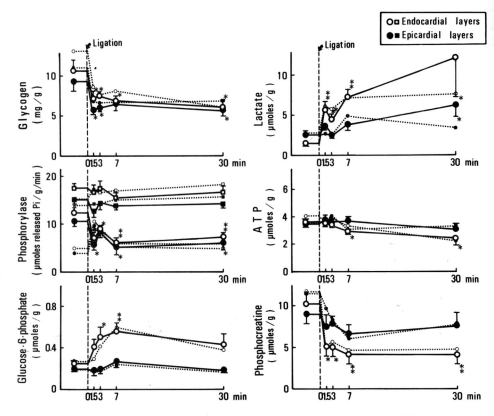

FIG. 7. Effect of pretreatment with carbochromen (4 mg/kg, i.v.) on the metabolic response to coronary artery ligation. Symbols are given in Figs. 2 and 3.

glycogenolytic and glycolytic processes (7). There is evidence that calcium ions activate phosphorylase by activating the phosphorylase b kinase (20). Therefore, it seems that calcium ions as well as catecholamines are functioning to regulate glycogenolysis in the myocardium.

Verapamil and nifedipine were reported to inhibit inward calcium current across the myocardial cell membrane (10). Accordingly, it is assumed that verapamil and nifedipine inhibit acceleration of glycogenolysis caused by coronary artery ligation.

In this series of experiments, therefore, verapamil or nifedipine was injected before coronary artery ligation. Verapamil (2.5 mg/ml; ample for injection, Eisai Co., Ltd.) was diluted with saline solution to make a solution of 200 μg/ml of verapamil, and nifedipine was first dissolved in absolute ethanol and next diluted with saline solution to a final concentration of 20 μg/ml of nifedipine in saline solution containing 1% ethanol. Since nifedipine is unstable when it is exposed to light, care was taken not to expose the drug during weighing, dissolving, and injecting. As a control for nifedipine, saline solution containing

1% ethanol was used. There were no significant differences, however, between the data obtained in saline-control experiments and ethanol-saline-control experiments.

Verapamil (100 μg/kg, i.v.) or nifedipine (10 μg/kg, i.v.) was injected 5 min before coronary artery ligation. After the injection of verapamil or nifedipine, heart rate increased slightly, and both systolic and diastolic blood pressures decreased rapidly and markedly. The decreased blood pressures returned to about 70 to 80% of the preinjection level within 5 min after the injection.

One of the most characteristic findings obtained in the nonischemic myocardium pretreated with verapamil was an increase in the activity of phosphorylase; the activity of phosphorylase a obtained 5 min after verapamil injection (endocardium, 9.99 $\pm$ 1.49; epicardium, 6.12 $\pm$ 0.87 μmoles released P_i/g/min) was higher than that obtained in the saline-control experiments (endocardium, 4.74 $\pm$ 0.28; epicardium, 3.94 $\pm$ 0.53 μmoles released P_i/g/min). The glycogen level in the verapamil experiments was lower than that obtained in the control experiments. The results regarding the activity of phosphorylase and the level of glycogen obtained in the nifedipine experiments were similar to those obtained in the verapamil experiments.

The metabolic response of the myocardium to coronary artery ligation in the presence of verapamil was also similar to the response in the presence of nifedipine. After coronary artery ligation, the activity of phosphorylase decreased, the G6P level increased, the lactate level increased, and the level of PCr decreased. The level of ATP did not change, even after coronary artery ligation. In general, there was no significant difference between the verapamil and nifedipine experiments.

The pattern of metabolic response to coronary artery ligation in the presence of verapamil or nifedipine is also similar to that in the presence of carbochromen. However, it is not clear why the activity of phosphorylase decreases after coronary artery ligation in dogs pretreated with verapamil, nifedipine, or carbochromen. Similar findings were also found in experiments with ouabain (1). In the experiments with verapamil, nifedipine, carbochromen, or ouabain, there is a common finding: The activity of phosphorylase increased after the drug injection alone. Therefore, it is possible to assume that the activity of phosphorylase does not increase further after coronary artery ligation because the activity of phosphorylase has been increased by the drug.

SUMMARY

In order to evaluate the action of antianginal drugs on the ischemic myocardium, the effect of pretreatment with antianginal drugs on the metabolic response to coronary artery ligation was studied. The levels of glycolytic intermediates, energy-rich phosphates, and the activity of phosphorylase were measured in the presence or absence of drugs and/or ischemia.

It was found that coronary artery ligation increased the activity of phosphorylase, elevated the levels of glycolytic intermediates, and decreased the level of PCr without affecting the ATP level. The increase in the activity of phosphorylase was inhibited by pretreatment with beta-adrenergic blocking agents such as propranolol and carteolol. Likewise, in the presence of nitroglycerin, coronary artery ligation did not increase the activity of phosphorylase. However, the mechanisms of the action of nitroglycerin and beta-adrenergic blocking agents seem to be different. In the presence of dipyridamole, the pattern of metabolic response to coronary artery ligation was not different from that obtained in the control experiments. Carbochromen, verapamil, or nifedipine increased the activity of phosphorylase. In the presence of carbochromen, verapamil, or nifedipine, the activity of phosphorylase decreased after coronary artery ligation. However, other metabolic responses of the myocardium to coronary artery ligation in the presence of carbochromen, verapamil, or nifedipine were similar to those obtained in the control experiments.

The metabolic response of the endocardium to ischemia was usually greater than that of the epicardial layers. It seems that the endocardial layers are more sensitive than the epicardial layers to coronary artery ligation. This finding was not modified by pretreatment with the drugs used in the present study.

In conclusion, the actions of nitroglycerin and beta-adrenergic blockers (propranolol and carteolol) seem to be similar when the myocardial metabolic response to ischemia is adopted as an index. The actions of carbochromen, verapamil, and nifedipine also seem to be similar, but they differ from the actions of nitroglycerin, propranolol, and carteolol.

REFERENCES

1. Abiko, Y., and Ichihara, K. (1978): Effect of ouabain on myocardial metabolic and contractile responses to coronary artery ligation. *Eur. J. Pharmacol.,* 47:87–94.
2. Abiko, Y., Minamidate, A., and Hashikawa, T. (1972): Discordant response to nitroglycerin of strain gauge arch and maximum rate of rise of left ventricular pressure in dogs. *Fukushima J. Med. Sci.,* 18:69–82.
3. Barker, S. B., and Summerson, H. (1941): The colorimetric determination of lactic acid in biological material. *J. Biol. Chem.,* 138:535–554.
4. Becker, L. C., Fortuin, N. J., and Pitt, B. (1971): Effect of ischemia and antianginal drugs on the distribution of radioactive microspheres in the canine left ventricle. *Circ. Res.,* 28:263–269.
5. Bergmeyer, H. U., editor (1974); *Methods of Enzymatic Analysis,* 2nd English ed. Academic Press, New York.
6. Cornblath, M., Randle, P. J., Parmeggiani, A., and Morgan, H. E. (1963): Regulation of glycogenolysis in muscle: Effects of glucagon and anoxia on lactate production, glycogen content, and phosphorylase activity in the perfused isolated rat heart. *J. Biol. Chem.,* 238:1592–1597.
7. Dhalla, N. S., Yates, J. C., and Proveda, V. (1977): Calcium-linked changes in myocardial metabolism in the isolated perfused rat heart. *Can. J. Physiol. Pharmacol.,* 55:925–933.
8. Fiske, C. H., and Subbarow, Y. (1925): The colorimetric determination of phosphorus. *J. Biol. Chem.,* 66:375–400.
9. Flameng, W., Schaper, W., and Lewi, P. (1973): Multiple experimental coronary occlusion without infarction. *Am. Heart J.,* 85:767–776.
10. Fleckenstein, A. (1971): Specific inhibitors and promoters of calcium action in the excitation–contraction coupling of heart muscle and their role in the prevention or production of myocardial

lesions. In: *Calcium and the Heart,* edited by P. Harris and L. H. Opie, pp. 135–188. Academic Press, New York.
11. Ichihara, K., and Abiko, Y. (1975): Difference between endocardial and epicardial utilization of glycogen in the ischemic heart. *Am. J. Physiol.,* 229:1585–1589.
12. Ichihara, K., and Abiko, Y. (1975): Effect of dipyridamole on the glycogen metabolism in the normal and ischemic canine myocardium. *Experientia,* 31:1198–1199.
13. Ichihara, K., and Abiko, Y. (1975): Glycogen metabolism and the effect of nitroglycerin on the glycogen metabolism in the normal and ischemic canine myocardium. *Experientia,* 31:477–478.
14. Ichihara, K., and Abiko, Y. (1977): Inhibition of endo- and epicardial glycogenolysis by propanolol in ischemic hearts. *Am. J. Physiol.,* 232:H349–H353.
15. Ichihara, K., Saitoh, Y., and Abiko, Y. (1977): Effect of carteolol, a new beta-adrenergic blocking agent, on myocardial metabolic response to coronary artery ligation in dogs. *Jpn. J. Pharmacol.,* 27:475–478.
16. Jedeikin, L. A. (1964): Regional distribution of glycogen and phosphorylase in the ventricles of the heart. *Circ. Res.,* 14:202–211.
17. Koyama, T., Scholtholt, J., and Nitz, R. E. (1972): The change of intramyocardial oxygen partial pressure after acute coronary occlusion and administration of carbochromen. *Arzneim. Forsch.,* 22:507–511.
18. Moir, T. W. (1972): Subendocardial distribution of coronary blood flow and the effect of antianginal drugs. *Circ. Res.,* 30:621–627.
19. Morgan, H. E., and Parmeggiani, A. (1964): Regulation of glycogenolysis in muscle: Effect of glucagon and anoxia on glycogenolysis in the perfused rat heart; effect of adenine nucleotides, glucose-6-phosphate and inorganic phosphate on muscle phosphorylase activity. *Ciba Found. Symp.,* pp. 254–272.
20. Namm, D. H., and Mayer, S. E. (1968): Effects of epinephrine on cardiac cyclic 3′,5′-AMP, phosphorylase kinase, and phosphorylase. *Mol. Pharmacol.,* 4:61–69.
21. Opie, L. H., (1968): Metabolism of the heart in health and disease. Part 1. *Am. Heart J.,* 76:685–698.
22. Opie, L. H. (1976): Effects of regional ischemia on metabolism of glucose and fatty acids. Relative rates of aerobic and anaerobic energy production during myocardial infarction and comparison with effect of anoxia. *Circ. Res. (Suppl. I),* 38:52–68.
23. Schraven, E., Trottnow, D., and Fiedler, V. B. (1976): Wirkung von Carbochromen auf Cyclisches Adenosinmonophosphat im Herzen. *Arzneim. Forsch.,* 26:200–204.
24. Seifter, S., Dayton, S., Novic, B., and Muntwyler, E. (1950): The determination of glycogen with the anthrone reagent. *Arch. Biochem. Biophys.,* 25:191–200.
25. Williamson, J. R. (1966): Glycolytic control mechanisms. II. Kinetics of intermediate changes during the aerobic–anaerobic transition in perfused rat heart. *J. Biol. Chem.,* 241:5026–5036.
26. Winbury, M. M., Howe, B. B., and Hefner, M. A. (1969): Effect of nitrates and other coronary dilators on large and small coronary vessels: An hypothesis for mechanism of action of nitrates. *J. Pharmacol. Exp. Ther.,* 168:70–95.
27. Winbury, M. M., Howe, B. B., and Weiss, H. R. (1971): Effect of nitroglycerin and dipyridamole on epicardial and endocardial oxygen tension—Further evidence for redistribution of myocardial blood flow. *J. Pharmacol. Exp. Ther.,* 176:184–199.
28. Wollenberger, A., and Shahab, L. (1965): Anoxia-induced release of noradrenaline from the isolated perfused heart. *Nature,* 270:88–89.
29. Yabuuchi, Y., and Kinoshita, D. (1974): Cardiovascular studies of 5-(3-tert-butylamino-2-hydroxy) propoxy-3,4-dihydrocarbostyril hydrochloride (OPC-1085), a new potent β-adrenergic blocking agent. *Jpn. J. Pharmacol.,* 24:853–861.

Ischemic Myocardium and Antianginal Drugs,
edited by M. M. Winbury and Y. Abiko.
Raven Press, New York © 1979.

New Experimental Models for the Development of Antianginal Drugs

W. Schaper

Max-Planck-Institute for Heart Research, Bad Nauheim, West Germany

The most important drugs used in the therapy of cardiac symptoms have been discovered by accident and are not the result of a planned pharmacologic experiment resting on a sound pathophysiologic basis. The usefulness of digitalis in dropsy and the effectiveness of nitroglycerin in angina pectoris are good examples of this statement. Ahlquist's receptor hypothesis, which he primarily designed to explain the complex actions of various natural and synthetic cate-cholamines in various organ systems, led finally to the development of beta-blocking drugs. But although beta blockers were developed in a much more direct and exclusively scientific way, they were not developed with the idea in mind to treat specific cardiac diseases. When these compounds became available, we just looked around for a suitable disease.

A REVIEW OF CURRENTLY USED MODELS FOR THE STUDY OF ANGINA AND INFARCTION

After the discovery of the beneficial effects of these compounds in angina pectoris, numerous animal experiments were carried out to find out if the damage of acute myocardial infarction could be minimized. The animal models used for this purpose showed a bewildering variation in the experimental setup, and it is difficult to draw conclusions with regard to the clinical situation.

In some experiments, the drugs were given before coronary occlusion; in other studies, they were given minutes after occlusion; and in still other studies, they were given a few hours after occlusion. Although these studies certainly establish the potential of the drugs under investigation, nothing can be said as to the therapeutic usefulness.

It follows from the foregoing that a therapeutic application of the compounds under study is much more meaningful, but this approach is hampered by our ignorance with regard to the time course of myocardial infarction and ischemia (i.e., by the unanswered question of how long it takes for reversible ischemia to develop into irreversible infarction). Studies with therapeutic application of a drug either use temporary coronary occlusion or permanent coronary occlusion. When temporary coronary occlusion is used, the ligature around the coronary artery is opened again and reflow is permitted. In this case, we are faced with the unsolved dilemma: Is reflow beneficial or detrimental? To my knowledge, determination of the effect of drugs administered some time after coronary occlusion, where occlusion remains permanent and infarct size is measured 24 to 48 hr after occlusion, has never been attempted, although this is the only clinically meaningful experiment. This experiment would require knowledge of the infarct size that would have developed without the experimental compound. This is difficult to obtain and requires a large control series because of the sizable scatter of infarct size.

The methods to produce ischemia also differ widely: Severe narrowing of a coronary artery, complete proximal occlusion, complete distal occlusion, distal occlusion of several branches, and combinations thereof have been described. All these models differ widely with regard to infarct size. If we consider that it is also important whether coronary occlusion was produced in awake animals or in an anesthetized preparation, whether the chest was open or closed, and whether heparin was or was not given, we arrive at a bewildering number of variables, which makes it very difficult to draw conclusions. My colleagues and I have studied most of these variables in our laboratory, and a short summary of our results follows:

(a) Severe narrowing of a coronary artery that preserves normal control flow with a normal myocardial oxygen consumption ($M\dot{V}O_2$) in an open chest situation is able to produce infarcts in the presence of very high oxygen consumption, i.e., with catecholamine stimulation.

(b) Proximal coronary artery occlusion, either permanent or longer than 2 hr, produces large infarcts.

(c) Distal small coronary artery occlusion produces very small and sometimes no infarcts.

(d) Distal occlusion of several small branches reduces collateral blood flow in the center of the combined areas; it produces a "twilight zone" of jeopardized myocardium around an infarcted core. Its clinical relevance is probably small because the experimental setup is very artificial.

(e) Studies in awake animals necessitate the previous implantation of measuring devices, such as flowmeters, catheters, occluders, and snares. Although results obtained from awake animals sound much more "physiologic," this method also has many disadvantages:
- The system is much more irritable.
- Parameters cannot be controlled.
- Animals have to be selected and trained.
- The chronic implantation of measuring devices decreases the fibrillation threshold and increases collateral blood flow because of the surgical handling of the heart.

This results in significantly smaller infarcts as compared to the anesthetized open chested dog.

(f) Infarcts can be produced in the anesthetized closed chest animal (dog) by catheter methods. Catheters are either wedged into coronary arteries, or they are used as carriers for occluding devices. Our experience with a catheter-guided gutta-percha plug[1] producing proximal left anterior descending coronary artery (LAD) occlusion showed the largest possible infarcts (i.e., the entire perfusion area of the occluded artery was necrotic 24 hr after occlusion).

We believe that the surgical preparation of a coronary artery leads to at least partial denervation and that plugging of that artery does not. It has not yet been proven that denervation produces reactions favoring smaller infarcts, but we think it to be likely.

MEASUREMENT OF INFARCT SIZE AND PERFUSION AREA

Although there is a plethora of papers dealing with infarct size, only very few have measured infarct size proper. Most investigators produce inferential evidence from markers of ischemia such as epicardial and precordial electrocardiograms, regional wall motion defects, or the release of enzymes.

Infarct size proper can be measured with great accuracy using histologic sections of the entire heart that are stained with hematoxylin and eosin. This is a very time-consuming method requiring technical skill, but it is the "gold standard" against which all other methods must be tested. Light microscopy requires that the animals live for about 24 to 48 hr after coronary occlusion, which is another reason why the "gold standard" is not very popular.

Still another problem is: When the size of an infarct is finally exactly measured, with what should it be compared? Most often, infarct size is expressed as a fraction of the entire left ventricle. This has serious disadvantages because the result is mainly dependent on the size of the occluded artery. I believe that it is much more meaningful to compare the size of an infarct to the perfusion area of the occluded coronary artery.

Frenzel, Hort, and I (1) devised the following method to define the perfusion area. After the experiment, the left coronary artery is cannulated with a ball-shaped cannula that is secured into the sinus of Valsalva with a purse-string suture. Barium sulfate gelatin is then injected under a pressure that is gradually increased from 75 mm Hg to 150 mm Hg within 6 min. The heart is then put into ice water until the injectate has gelled; thereafter, the heart is sliced into 1-cm-thick slices. X-Ray arteriograms of these slices are then prepared by exposing the slices (on fine-grained film) to 20 kV at 30 mA (i.e., "soft" X-rays). There are several ways to define the area of perfusion from each slice angiogram:

(a) The angle of penetration into the myocardium of coronary sub-branches differs between the LAD and left circumflex (LC) sub-branches.
(b) The bed of the ligated artery does not fill with contrast medium.
(c) Only the epicardial branches of the occluded artery were injected with

---

[1] M. Gottwik and J. Ashkenazi, *personal communication.*

barium and not the small endomural vessels. The difference between the injected vasculature of the adjacent normal tissue and that of the infarcted tissue is like the difference between a "summer tree" and a "winter tree."

After the area of perfusion of the occluded artery is defined on a slice of myocardium, this area is measured by planimetry and compared with the area of infarction.

The slice of myocardium from which we measured the perfusion area is also used for the determination of infarct size by histology. The entire slice is cut (after it is fixed and embedded in paraffin) on a large microtome, and after it is stained, the infarcted zone is drawn on the section while it is viewed with the light microscope. Great caution must be taken in these procedures to ensure that the angiographed slice and the histologic section taken from it do not differ in size because one image is projected over the other. This technique is extremely time consuming, and we have therefore developed a similar but much quicker method from which all the information is available at the end of one working day. The modification consists of replacing histology with selective dehydrogenase staining using tetrazolium salts. These methods are long known; they are used routinely in autopsy diagnosis, but the application to experimental infarcts proved difficult because the addition of succinate as a substrate did not produce differential staining in the dog heart. This constitutes a species difference; i.e., in experimental canine infarction, succinic dehydrogenase does not leave the infarcted myocardium nor is it inactivated. When malate or lactate are used as substrates, a very clear demarcation between infarcted and noninfarcted tissue is seen. We use malate routinely as a substrate because it has the added advantage that excess malate inhibits succinic dehydrogenase.

We then compared histologic infarct size with macrohistochemic infarct size using two experimental designs. The LAD was permanently ligated in anesthetized dogs who were sacrificed 48 hr after ligation. The hearts were randomly assigned to either a group to be studied histologically or a group to be studied macrohistochemically. The histologic investigation was done in the Department of Pathology, University of Marburg, West Germany (Prof. Hort), and the macrohistochemical group was processed in our laboratory. The agreement between methods was excellent: 72% of the perfusion area was histologically infarcted and 74.5% was macrohistochemically infarcted. Thereafter, the macrohistochemically diagnosed group was also studied histologically; i.e., the para nitrobluetetrazolium (p-NBT)-stained borders were studied histologically, and an excellent agreement within the same heart was found.

Although permanent occlusion is the best imaginable test for the study of myocardial protection, it is impracticable because the flow of data is too slow. Two observations considerably shortened the procedure:

(a) We found that, at a normal $M\dot{V}O_2$ of 8 ml/min/100 g, 80% of the final infarct size was already obtained after 90 min of coronary occlusion.

(b) When ischemic tissue is reperfused after 90 min of occlusion, staining with p-NBT results much earlier in a discrimination between infarcted and noninfarcted zones. After 60 min of reperfusion, a clear delineation of the infarct is visible.

The rapid quantitative diagnosis of infarcts 60 min after reflow is not possible with any other method.

THE "DOUBLE-VESSEL" MODEL

Our technique enabled us to design acute intervention studies within the same heart. This was achieved by occluding two medium-sized coronary sub-branches in succession—one to produce a control infarct and the other to study the effect of an intervention on a "test" infarct. First, a medium-sized artery is occluded for 90 min, whereafter the area is reperfused. After quieting from possible arrhythmias (usually not longer than 15 min), the second artery is occluded and simultaneously the intervention is started. Also 90 min later, the test artery is reperfused for another 90 min. Thereafter, the heart is excised, and the coronaries are filled with $BaSO_4$ gelatin, sliced, and incubated in p-NBT-malate. The stained slices are photographed on color transparency film. Both infarcts are then compared with the respective perfusion areas and with each other.

In order to establish validation criteria for this new model, we designed and carried out the following experiments: (a) simultaneous occlusion and reperfusion of both coronary arteries to see if both infarcts are of equal size when occluded under identical hemodynamic conditions; and (b) sequential occlusion and reperfusion of both arteries to find out if mild hemodynamic differences that naturally exist between the two occlusion periods significantly affect infarct size.

We found that under both conditions (i.e., simultaneous and sequential occlusion), both infarcts were of equal size as compared to their respective areas of risk. We found, however, that both arteries had to be of equal size within narrow limits; i.e., they had to perfuse a territory of equal size. We found an inverse correlation between the area of risk and collateral blood flow; i.e., large areas of ischemia receive relatively little collateral blood flow and vice versa. This again correlated well with the finding that the size of the ensuing infarct grows with the size of the area at risk.

CONCLUSION

We designed a new model for experimental myocardial infarction intervention studies based on the principle of double coronary artery occlusion. One coronary artery is occluded under control conditions, the other under intervention conditions. This new method necessitates finite occlusion time for both arteries for a clear separation between control and intervention. Ninety minutes of occlusion followed by reflow is a suitable time interval. Reperfusion facilitates early macro-histochemical diagnosis of infarct size, probably because of the rapid washout of enzymes from irreversibly damaged cells. Infarcts are first expressed as the necrotic fraction of the area at risk and then compared with each other.

REFERENCE

1. Schaper, W., Frenzel, J., and Hort, W. (1979): Experimental coronary artery occlusion. I. Measurement of infarct size. *Basic Res. Cardiol.,* 74:46–53.

Ischemic Myocardium and Antianginal Drugs,
edited by M. M. Winbury and Y. Abiko.
Raven Press, New York © 1979.

Discussion: Antianginal Drugs

Martin M. Winbury, *Chairman*

Winbury: I will start with Dr. Abiko. In your slide on the changes in glycogen following coronary occlusion, there was a drop, a rise, and then a gradual decline. What is the significance of those changes?

Abiko: I suppose that glycogenolysis was accelerated immediately after ischemia and then inhibited, probably because of an inhibition of the breakdown of glycogen and an increase in the synthesis of glycogen. The metabolic response to ischemia is not a constant one, but it is regulated by many factors. For example, an increase in glycogenolysis will produce a high concentration of G6P in the tissue, and the increase in G6P will accelerate synthesis of glycogen, leading to a decreased rate of breakdown of glycogen.

Winbury: The other thing that I get out of your presentation is that nitroglycerin was different from other drugs in providing some protection. We heard from Dr. Bing that nitroglycerin has no direct metabolic effect. Would your studies be interpreted as indicating an indirect or a direct metabolic effect?

Abiko: I really cannot answer that question. But the action of nitroglycerin on metabolism is probably not a result of a direct effect because there is no evidence of direct action on metabolism, as mentioned by Dr. Bing.

Bleifeld: Dr. Henry, do you recommend the use of calcium antagonists in patients with preinfarction angina who will be operated on?

Henry: Well, we have not done any clinical studies. As you know, the variability of the natural history of unstable angina makes therapeutic trials very difficult, and we have thus far not used the drug to treat preinfarction angina. However, recent work in Japan suggests that widespread use of nifedipine and diltiazem may reduce the prevalence of unstable angina in patients suffering from coronary heart disease. These observations have not yet been confirmed.

Bleifeld: My question refers to protection during the operation.

Henry: During ischemic standstill, one has the best situation to assess ischemic injury. Our studies in dogs were sufficiently encouraging for Dr. Clark to initiate at our institution a trial in patients. However, we do not have enough observations to make a statement about the efficacy of nifedipine cardioplegia in man.

Opie: Sorry. That is not exactly the condition Dr. Bleifeld was talking about. Dr. Bleifeld was referring to patients with preinfarction angina. So you cannot necessarily extrapolate from Dr. Henry's conditions to Dr. Bleifeld's conditions.

Bleifeld: Well, people who have preinfarction angina or unstable angina have a high risk in bypass surgery. So I asked if Dr. Henry recommends calcium antagonists to reduce that risk.

Opie: May I continue on that point? Do you know the cause of preinfarction angina? If one does not know the basic mechanism, then one does not necessarily know whether calcium antagonists are acting to protect during the operative period or acting on the coronary arteries.

Bing: It bothers me that we know a lot about what metabolic changes take place during infarction, but the only thing we know about angina, whether it is preinfarction or otherwise, is that there is a rise in end-diastolic pressure and that the heart really goes into failure. But I do not know of any studies that show that in angina any metabolic effect takes place.

Henry: One of the problems in evaluating coronary bypass surgery is that, in the surgical literature, the incidence of acute myocardial infarction after bypass surgery is anywhere between 5 and 30%, and the criteria that have been used to assess myocardial infarction are just not solid. However, it is undisputed that a previous infarction constitutes an important risk factor in coronary disease.

Opie: When we say failure of medical treatment, generally we mean failure of nitrates and beta blockade to work; however, unless calcium antagonist agents have been tried as well, one cannot say that medical treatment has failed. In angina at rest, Maseri of Pisa has shown that the EKG changes precede the changes in the left ventricular function. However, in angina of effort, the first change involves failure of the heart.

Winbury: When you talk of angina at rest that does not respond to conventional therapy, do you mean vasospasm? I thought that Maseri shows relief of vasospasm by nitrates.

Opie: It is quite true that nitrates and calcium antagonists work in so-called vasospastic angina. Maseri makes the point that it is possible that spasm contributes to preinfarction angina or to angina at rest. If spasm is a calcium-mediated phenomenon, then one can say that treatment has not worked if one has also tried calcium antagonists. But there are no control studies on this. The number of studies even showing that beta blockade works in preinfarction angina is very limited.

Nakamura: May I add a few words regarding Dr. Opie's question and comment? We have clinical experience with Japanese patients who are suffering from effort and rest angina. I do not have experience with or know of a case that shows a dramatic effect of calcium antagonists in relieving angina. We feel that, in terms of relieving angina attacks, nitroglycerin is more clearly effective, even when patients respond to calcium antagonists as well. We had a single blind crossover study (drug, placebo, and drug) and, from this study, we reached that conclusion.

Winbury: Dr. Nakamura, regarding diltiazem, you suggested that there was an improvement in the epicardial perfusion in ischemic region, but not in the endocardial perfusion. Now, what do you feel then is the mechanism of effectiveness, if diltiazem is effective? My first question is whether diltiazem is effective in angina of effort or primarily in Prinzmetal vasospastic, and, if it is effective in angina of effort, what is the mechanism?

Nakamura: Are you asking if diltiazem is effective in angina of effort?

Winbury: Yes, do you find it effective in angina of effort?

Nakamura: No, I am not convinced of it yet.

Winbury: It relieves Prinzmetal angina or angina at rest. What is the mechanism there?

Nakamura: I am not sure, but probably it is due to release of spasm.

Winbury: Now wasn't there some work coming from this country that also implicated alpha-adrenergic mechanisms because someone showed that phentolamine was effective 4 or 5 years ago. Is that right? Who is the author?

Nakamura: It is not me. When we talk about variant angina or rest angina, it is very difficult to evaluate the drug effect because of the large scattering of variation in frequency and incidence of occurrence. For example, a patient who has 20 attacks a day will have no attacks in the next week without any medication. Therefore, it is very difficult to establish reproducibility. Therefore, regarding phentolamine or other drugs, I cannot make any comments at present.

W. Schaper: I would like to ask Dr. Abiko a question. I noticed that your nucleotide data are very stable. Coming back to my own presentation, I noticed that you occluded a sub-branch of the left anterior descending coronary artery. Now, I would expect that you have 20 ml/min of collateral flow. Could it be that the stable levels of nucleotides can be ascribed to this "hypo-ischemia?"

Abiko: If the ischemic area is more extensive, the ATP level will decrease after ischemia. The reason why we ligated the small branch is that, if we ligate the major branch, arrhythmias will occur and the arrhythmias will probably affect myocardial metabolism.

Hashimoto: Dr. Abiko, was the increase in the phosphorylase activity produced by drugs significant?

Abiko: Yes. When we injected nifedipine, verapamil, or carbochromen, activity of phosphorylase a was increased. The reason for this is not clear, but there is a paper reporting that carbochromen increases the myocardial cyclic AMP level. This might be responsible for the increase in phosphorylase activity induced by carbochromen.

Hashimoto: Which is more important, glycogen level or phosphorylase activity, for the evaluation of metabolic data?

Abiko: The activity of phosphorylase is more important. According to Dr. Wollenberger, catecholamine release occurs after myocardial ischemia. This leads to an increase in the phosphorylase activity and then to a decrease in the glycogen level.

Bleifeld: I would like to ask Dr. Schaper a question. You showed that a delayed infarct developed in the subgroup of medium-sized myocardial oxygen consumption and relatively high flow. But the final infarct size was the same as that in the other group. Furthermore, you showed infarction during propranolol. Is that not in disagreement with the other groups?

W. Schaper: No, it is not in disagreement because the infarct size under beta-adrenergic blockade was for just a 90-min period of occlusion. You know, in our two-vessel model, we occluded just two times in 90 min. On the graph, this is 2 hr at least, and it is then compared with the permanent occlusion.

Bleifeld: In conclusion, propranolol does nothing after 2 hr?

W. Schaper: Well, I would say it delays the irreversible injury for up to 6 hr. However, the final infarct size is not affected, that is, infarct size after 24 or 48 hr. If you continue treatment over this period of time, the final infarct size is not different from an untreated population.

Bing: Dr. Schaper, the basis for nitrobluetetrazolium activity is an NAD–NADH reaction. Is it not a hydrogen acceptor?

W. Schaper: Yes, that is true.

Bing: So, as the infarct occurs, an excess of reduced nicotinamide adenine dinucleotides will be there. Is that what the basis of the reaction is? I mean NADH will be in excess because it is not being converted into NAD. That must be the fundamental mechanism of the reaction, which means that a lot of reduced equivalents are floating around at the same time. I am just trying to think of the biochemistry. The other thing that I want to ask about is the question of the border zone. When I look at your slide, I do not see much of the "twilight zone" here. There seems to be a rather sharp division between the infarcted and the noninfarcted area. Is that correct?

W. Schaper: That is absolutely correct. The border zone to me is an amount of epicardium that can be salvaged. But there is no lateral border. The border is very sharp.

Bing: Well this, as you know, is the bone of contention among many people. Dr. Opie is one of them and Dr. Britton Chance another. I think Britton Chance did find a sharp demarcation line. Is that not right, Lionel?

Opie: Who are you questioning?

Bing: Britton Chance, not you.

Opie: I will come back to this point later because Chance's concept of the on–off metabolism of the mitochondria, that it is functioning either flat-out or not at all, is a very interesting point. But to carry on with comments made by Dr. Bing, may I ask Dr. Schaper a question about the comparison of the biochemical criterion, NBT, with the histological criterion? Was that histological criterion taken at the same time, that is to say, after 90 min of occlusion, or was it taken 48 hr later? I did not quite get that point.

W. Schaper: Well, we did several validation studies. We ligated a coronary artery permanently, stained it, and sent the stained slides to Professor Hort. He photographed this and then sectioned it by large microtome and compared histological infarct size with the nitroblue stain area.

Opie: But the data you presented here were based on 90 min.

W. Schaper: Yes.

Opie: Now did you compare 90 min of NADH accumulation with the gold standard, your 48-hr tissue necrosis? Or did you compare NADH at 48 hr with the gold standard at 48 hr?

W. Schaper: We did two more validation studies. We had 90 min of occlusion, followed by reperfusion. The animal lived for two more days, and then we compared histology and the nitrobluetetrazolium. This compared very favorably. But we still felt that this procedure was too long, so we then tried 90 min of occlusion followed by 90 min of reperfusion to obtain all the data in one working day. In this case, of course, the data are getting a little more "soft" because, after 90 min of occlusion and 90 min of reperfusion, the pathologist is less secure in his diagnosis. We have two points of evidence here. The good agreement between histology and staining prompted us to accept the data at face value. Nevertheless, we sent these 90-min-occlusion–90-min-reperfusion samples to the pathologist and asked him if he could predict infarct size. He found that he could, simply by looking at the waviness of the myocyte, which probably had not contracted but had expanded ununiformly so that it appeared in the light microscope as a waviness of fibers. This is a symptom that has been described by Hort. This is accepted as a sign of irreversible damage. However, to me, these data are a lot softer than the 2-day data.

Opie: I would like to ask you just one further question. If there is, then, a good relation between 90-min NADH and ultimate histology, why did you say that propranolol reduced 90-min infarct size but did not reduce 2-day infarct size? Did I understand that correctly?

W. Schaper: When you study a 90-min occlusion period under the influence of beta-adrenergic blocking agents, you find a small infarction, according to our criteria. If you have a permanent occlusion under the influence of beta-adrenergic blocking agents or whatever agents you use to decrease myocardial oxygen consumption, the final infarct size is not different from that of a non-treated population.

Opie: But does that not then suggest that 90-min infarct size is not a reflection of your 2-day infarct size?

W. Schaper: Of course not; it is just a delay. We have ischemia here but not necrosis; however, necrosis eventually develops. What is gained during these 90 min is lost in the ensuing 22 hr.

Bing: One thing that I understand now is that necrosis is really a slowly progressing histological process, but the tetrazolium is an immediate situation in which the NADH and NAD relationship is expressed.

Winbury: What is the significance of protection at 90 min in relation to this procedure as a new model for antianginal drugs? I can see that you have a comparison of an untreated area subjected to catecholamines with an area protected by beta blockers, but ultimately you get the same end effect. Are you suggesting that the 90-min effect indicates that there is some protection?

But actually, there is no real protection because you will still go on to get the same size of infarct. Several of us are confused about that.

W. Schaper: Well, to give you the message in very basic terms, I do not believe in the concept of reducing infarct size.

Winbury: I am 100% in accord with you on that. I think we agree there. Then we would say that this model still does not indicate whether a compound is or is not an antianginal agent.

W. Schaper: That, of course, is totally different. You can treat ischemia as long as you have all the circumstances that can make it reversible; that is, if you restore flow in due time, everything is fine. I think there is merit in using these compounds that delay final necrosis because we can envisage that our treatment of patients with very early myocardial infarction can be improved by using more aggressive methods—that is, by assisting circulation and then by somehow establishing blood flow.

Winbury: I think that this provocative discussion has to end now, and I will give the chair to Dr. Bing.

Metabolic Changes

Ischemic Myocardium and Antianginal Drugs,
edited by M. M. Winbury and Y. Abiko.
Raven Press, New York © 1979.

Energy Metabolism in Ischemic Myocardium As Studied in the Isolated Perfused Guinea Pig Heart

Shoichi Imai, Yumi Katano, Norio Shimamoto, and Ken Sakai

Department of Pharmacology, Niigata University School of Medicine, Niigata 951, Japan

As stated by Bing et al. (3), mammalian cardiac muscle function is exquisitely sensitive to oxygen. In its absence, mechanical performance declines rapidly and persisting function and subsequent integrity of myocardial tissue are compromised. A number of factors influencing the viability of ischemic heart muscle have been examined (17), and it has been suggested that the ability of the heart to survive and recover from periods of inadequate oxygenation depends upon sufficient reserves of energy-rich phosphates remaining available to maintain cellular function and membrane integrity (12,15).

The purpose of the present study was to characterize the changes in the myocardial energy-rich phosphate compounds produced by total coronary occlusion for varying lengths of time. Particular attention was directed toward the reversibility of these metabolic derangements. Understanding of the maximal period of coronary occlusion and of the characteristic metabolic derangements that are compatible with reversibility of ischemic injury upon reperfusion is essential for development of methods to salvage ischemic myocardium and for successful treatment of myocardial infarction in man.

MATERIALS AND METHODS

Experiments were performed in the isolated perfused heart preparation of the guinea pig (Langendorff's preparation). Guinea pigs of either sex weighing between 300 and 500 g were sacrificed by a blow on the head. Immediately after opening the thorax, the hearts were rapidly excised and transferred to ice-chilled Krebs–Ringer solution to induce rapid cessation of the heartbeat, after which they were dissected from the mediastinum. The ascending aorta was cannulated and retrograde perfusion with a modified Krebs–Ringer bicarbonate solution from a reservoir 75 cm above the heart was begun immediately. The perfusion fluid contained NaCl (127.2 mM), KCl (4.7 mM), $CaCl_2$ (2.5 mM), KH_2PO_4 (1.2 mM), and $NaHCO_3$ (24.9 mM). It was doubly aerated with 95% O_2 + 5% CO_2 to ensure Po_2 values higher than 600 mm Hg and kept at a temperature of 38 ± 0.3°C. Sodium pyruvate (2.0 mM) and glucose (5.5 mM) were added to the perfusion solution as substrates. The preparation was placed in a moist chamber, which was also kept at a temperature of 38 ± 0.3°C, and was allowed to equilibrate for 1 hr. A cannulating-type probe (1.5 mm i.d.) of an electromagnetic flowmeter (Stathum SP 2201) placed just in front of the aortic cannula measured the mean coronary inflow. The heart rate was taken from either the perfusion or the left ventricular isovolumetric pressure pulses. Left ventricular isovolumetric pressure was recorded with a flaccid saline-filled urethane polymer balloon (Takeda Chemical Ind.) that was connected to a pressure transducer (Nihon Kohden LPU 0.5) with polyethylene tubing. The first derivative of the left ventricular pressure was obtained with an electronic differentiator with a time constant of 5 msec (San-ei Sokki). The maximum rate of the rise of systolic pressure *(dp/dt_{max})* was obtained from the recording of the first derivative of ventricular pressure and was used as an index of the inotropic state of the heart. According to Furnival et al. (10), this is a more reliable index of inotropic changes in the ventricle than peak pressure in the left ventricle, duration of systole, or stroke work at constant end-diastolic pressure. An electromagnetic oscilloscope (Yokogawa Electric Works Photocorder 2924) and a linearly recording ink-writing oscillograph (Watanabe Instruments WTR 281) were the recording systems used. Hearts that did not fulfill the following criteria after the equilibration period of 30 min were discarded: spontaneous heart rate above 200/min and at least doubling of coronary flow on release of a 30-sec period of inflow occlusion.

At the end of the experimental period, the hearts were rapidly excised and immediately frozen with a pair of Wollenberger tongs precooled in liquid N_2. The frozen tissue fragments were reduced to a fine powder in a stainless steel percussion mortar (13) cooled in liquid N_2 and then homogenized with 2 volumes of 0.6 N perchloric acid (PCA) at 0°C. After centrifugation with a refrigerated centrifuge (3,000 rpm for 15 min), the residue was homogenized again with 2 volumes of 0.2 N PCA and centrifuged. The combined supernatant was neutralized with 5 N KOH. Adenine nucleotides were separated by the thin-layer chromatographic (TLC) method of Jones et al. (14) by using polyethyleneimine (PEI)-impregnated cellulose plates and were quantitated directly on the plates by UV absorption with a dual-wavelength TLC scanner (Shimadzu CS-900). Total phosphate contents [inorganic phosphate (P_i) plus creatine phosphate] were determined by the method of Fiske and Subbarow (9) by incubating an aliquot of the neutralized muscle extract with the acid–molybdate reagent for 30 min at 25°C. Creatine phosphate was determined on a second aliquot after all the inorganic phosphates were precipitated with alkaline $CaCl_2$ (pH 9), according to the method described by Fawaz and Fawaz (7).

In order to assess the energy status of the myocardium, the phosphorylation potential (Γ) was calculated using the following equation:

$$\Gamma = \frac{[ATP]}{[ADP][P_i]},$$

where ATP represents adenosine triphosphate and ADP, adenosine diphosphate.

According to Lehninger (16), this is a sensitive indicator of the energy status of a cell: the higher the phosphorylation potential, the more highly "energized" the cell.

Atkinson and Walton's energy charge (1) was also calculated:

$$\text{Energy charge} = \frac{[\text{ATP}] + \frac{1}{2}[\text{ADP}]}{[\text{ATP}] + [\text{ADP}] + [\text{AMP}]},$$

where AMP represents adenosine monophosphate.

Myocardial lactate content was determined by a spectrophotometric method with lactic dehydrogenase, as described in a previous publication (19). Pyruvate content was determined with a fluorimetric method of Passonneau and Lowry (20). On the basis of these determinations, the myocardial redox potential *(Eh)* was calculated using the following equation (11):

$$Eh \text{ (mV)} = -204 - 30.7 \log \frac{\text{lactate content}}{\text{pyruvate content}}.$$

In order to get information about the release of lactate from the heart, samples of the perfusion medium (6 to 8 ml) were collected in the ice-chilled test tubes at different time intervals during the experimental time period, and the lactate concentration was determined. Lactate output was calculated by multiplying the lactate concentration thus obtained by the corresponding coronary flow.

RESULTS

Energy Status of the Isolated Perfused Guinea Pig Heart

Myocardial high-energy phosphate levels determined *in situ* in hearts of anesthetized animals are listed in the left-hand column in Table 1. Animals were anesthetized by intraperitoneal administration of urethane (1.0 g/kg). Under artificial respiration with air, the thorax was opened and the heart exposed. After an equilibration period of 30 min, the hearts were quickly excised and frozen with Wollenberger tongs precooled in liquid N_2.

TABLE 1. *Concentration of high-energy phosphates of the isolated guinea pig heart*

High-energy phosphate[a]	*In situ* ($n = 4$)	1-hr perfusion ($n = 11$)
ATP	3.73 ± 0.18	3.54 ± 0.14
ADP	0.71 ± 0.02	0.82 ± 0.06
AMP	0.14 ± 0.01	0.16 ± 0.03
CP	4.02 ± 0.36	4.30 ± 0.17
P_i	4.25 ± 0.30	4.07 ± 0.45

[a] Measured in μmoles/g wet weight.

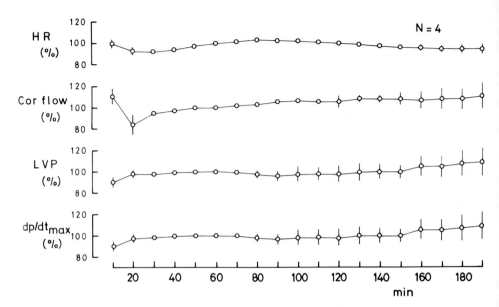

FIG. 1. Mechanical performances of the isolated perfused heart preparation of the guinea pig. HR, heart rate per minute expressed as a percentage of the value attained after the equilibration period of 1 hr; Cor flow, coronary inflow expressed as a percentage of the value attained after the equilibration period of 1 hr; LVP, left ventricular pressure expressed as a percentage of the value attained after the equilibration period of 1 hr; dp/dt$_{max}$, the maximum rate of rise of the left ventricular pressure expressed as a percentage of the value attained after the equilibration period of 1 hr.

The values of HR, Cor flow, LVP, and dp/dt$_{max}$ attained after the equilibration period of 1 hr were 241.3 ± 10.5/min, 8.4 ± 1.4 ml/min, 59.7 ± 3.0 mm Hg, and 1,001 ± 98.2 mm Hg/sec, respectively.

The right-hand column in Table 1 illustrates the myocardial high-energy phosphate levels of the isolated perfused hearts, determined after an equilibration period of 1 hr. As is evident from Table 1, the myocardial energy status of the isolated perfused hearts supplied with glucose plus pyruvate does not deviate significantly from that of the *in situ* heart.

Corresponding to the maintenance of the physiological state of myocardial energy metabolism, the hemodynamic parameters were also within the physiological range for more than 3 hr, as shown in Fig. 1. The autoregulation of the coronary vasculature was well maintained, and the reactivity of the coronary system as judged by a reactive hyperemic response was essentially unchanged during the entire course of the experimental period.

Effects of Ischemia on the Myocardial Content of High-Energy Phosphate Compounds

Figures 2 and 3 illustrate the changes in the myocardial content of high-energy phosphate compounds produced by occlusion of the coronary inflow

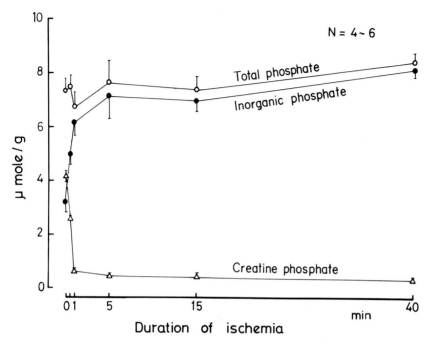

FIG. 2. Effects of ischemia of varying length on the myocardial content of total phosphate, creatine phosphate, and inorganic phosphate.

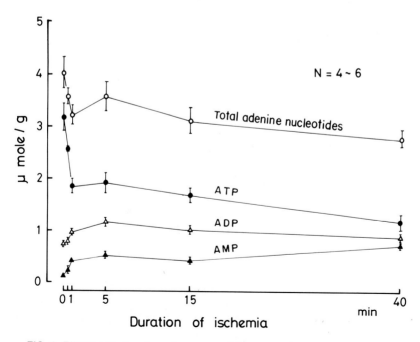

FIG. 3. Effects of ischemia on the myocardial content of adenine nucleotides.

for varying lengths of time. Breakdown of the creatine phosphate proceeded very rapidly; it was almost completely depleted within 1 min of ischemia, and no further decrease was noted with longer ischemia. The decline of ATP content was very rapid during the first minute of ischemia, leveled off for a while, and then accelerated again after 15 min. Figure 4 depicts the relationship between the myocardial content of creatine phosphate and ATP following occlusion of the coronary artery. The differential depletion of creatine phosphate and ATP demonstrated in Fig. 4 is in accord with a kinetic heterogeneity of ATP and creatine phosphate breakdown, as reported by Gudbjarnason et al. (12). The P_i content increased as a mirror image to the decrease in creatine phosphate, while AMP increased as a mirror image to the decrease in ATP. ADP content increased. Whereas there was a slight gradual rise of the total phosphate content, a diminution of the total adenine nucleotide content was noted. As shown in Fig. 5, energy charge decreased, reflecting a decrease in ATP content, whereas phosphorylation potential decreased in parallel with the changes in creatine phosphate.

Figure 6 illustrates the changes in the mechanical performances of the heart induced by an abrupt cessation of the coronary flow. As is demonstrated in this figure, there was a precipitous fall in the left ventricular systolic pressure and in the maximum rate of development of the left ventricular pressure. After 1 min, both were less than 50% of the initial value. Complete loss of contractile

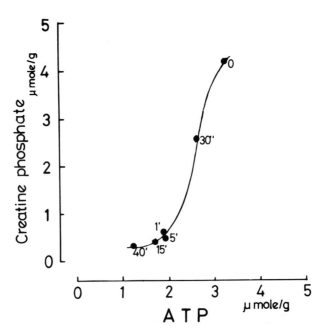

FIG. 4. Relationship between the myocardial content of creatine phosphate and ATP following occlusion of coronary inflow.

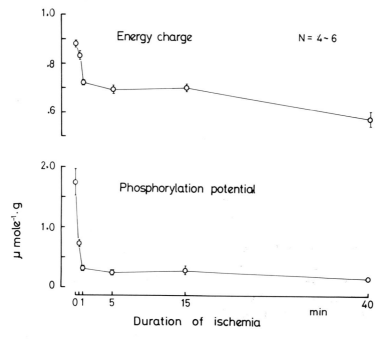

FIG. 5. Effects of ischemia on the phosphorylation potential and the energy charge.

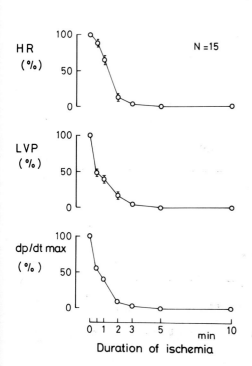

FIG. 6. Effects of ischemia on the mechanical performances of the heart. HR, heart rate per minute expressed as a percentage of the preocclusion value; LVP, left ventricular systolic pressure expressed as a percentage of the preocclusion value; dp/dt_{max}, the maximum rate of rise of the left ventricular pressure expressed as a percentage of the preocclusion value; The preocclusion values of HR, LVP, and dp/dt_{max} were 226.8 ± 4.66/min, 60.6 ± 1.36 mm Hg, and $1,132.6 \pm 84.88$ mm Hg/sec, respectively ($n = 15$).

activity was noted with ischemia of 3 min duration or longer. The heart rate decreased. However, the changes in the heart rate proceeded relatively slowly during the initial 1-min period.

Effects of Ischemia on Myocardial Lactate and Pyruvate

As shown in Fig. 7, there was a definite accumulation of lactate in the myocardium, which increased with longer occlusion. Since pyruvate content decreased, the redox potential of the myocardium *(Eh)* changed to more negative values.

Effects of Reperfusion

After occlusions of the coronary inflow of varying lengths of time, perfusion was resumed, and the recovery of the energy-rich phosphate compounds was examined.

As illustrated in Fig. 8, after a 1-min ischemic period, there was an almost complete restitution of ATP during the first 30-min period of reperfusion, which was followed by a secondary decline to a level of around 60% of the preocclusion value. After occlusions of longer duration (i.e., 5 and 15 min), restitution of ATP was observed only during the first 15-min period of reperfusion. After

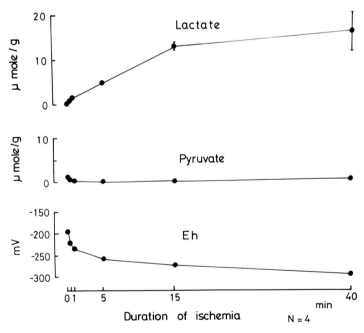

FIG. 7. Effects of ischemia on the myocardial content of lactate and pyruvate and on the myocardial redox potential (Eh).

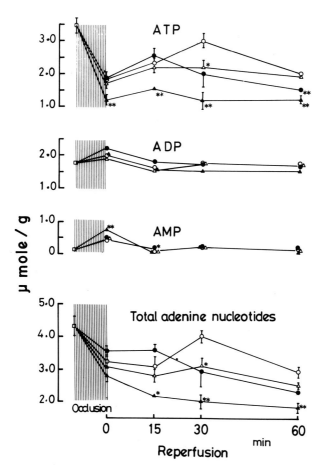

FIG. 8. Effects of reperfusion after occlusion of coronary inflow on the myocardial content of adenine nucleotides. *Open circles,* 1 min; *solid circles,* 5 min; *open triangles,* 15 min; *solid triangles,* 40 min. Student's *t*-test was applied using the method for unpaired observations. Significant differences against the corresponding values for 1 min of occlusion: *, $p < 0.05$; **, $p < 0.01$.

occlusions of the longest duration used (i.e., 40 min), the ATP level was significantly lower at any time during the recovery process than those of the recovery periods following shorter occlusions. In contrast, the restitution of ADP and AMP content was found to be almost complete. As shown in Fig. 9, recovery of the creatine phosphate was quite marked during the first 15-min period of reperfusion. However, the higher level was not maintained, and the creatine phosphate content declined to around 60% of the preocclusion level. Restitution of the P_i content was complete after 15 min of reperfusion. These findings are in agreement with those obtained by Coffman et al. (5), Benson et al. (2), and Feinstein (8).

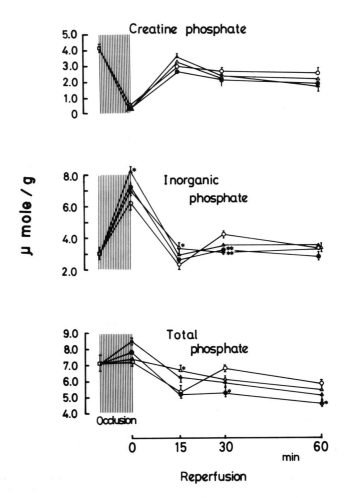

FIG. 9. Effects of reperfusion after occlusion of coronary inflow on the myocardial content of creatine phosphate, inorganic phosphate, and total phosphate. Symbols are given in Fig. 8.

Despite the incomplete restoration of ATP, the energy charge, after slight initial fluctuations, regained the values around 0.8, independent of the duration of the preceding ischemic period, as shown in Fig. 10. The restitution of the phosphorylation potential also proceeded with an initial fluctuation before finally reaching values around 40 to 60% of the preocclusion level (Fig. 10).

Associated with the accumulation of lactate during the ischemic period was a release of this substance into the perfusate upon reperfusion, and a close relation was noted between the amount of lactate accumulated within the myocardium during the ischemic period and the amount released just after reperfusion (Fig. 11). A complete reversal of lactate accumulation was observed after

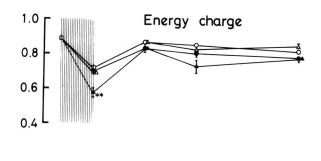

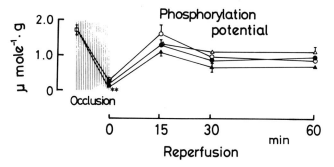

FIG. 10. Effects of reperfusion after occlusion of coronary inflow on the phosphorylation potential and the energy charge. Symbols are given in Fig. 8.

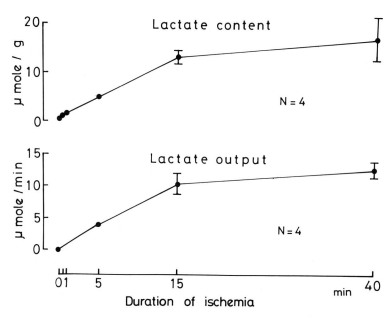

FIG. 11. The lactate output from the heart that occurred on reperfusion as related to the amount of lactate accumulated within the myocardium after occlusions of varying lengths of time.

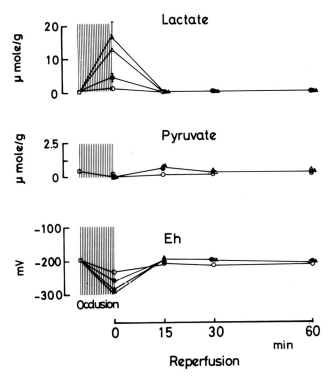

FIG. 12. Effects of reperfusion after occlusion of coronary inflow on the myocardial content of lactate, pyruvate, and the myocardial redox potential (Eh). Symbols are given in Fig. 8.

15 min of reperfusion, independent of the duration of the preceding ischemia, as shown in Fig. 12.

As shown in Fig. 13, the mechanical performances of the heart were restored almost completely upon reperfusion, even after 40 min of ischemia.

DISCUSSION

One of the purposes of the present study was to characterize the metabolic derangements produced by ischemic insult and to assess the reversibility of these derangements. While the depletion of creatine phosphate content was almost instantaneous, three distinct phases were noted in the process of depletion of ATP. Without doubt, the first phase—a rapid decline—was brought about by a sudden cessation of oxidative production of this compound in the face of almost normal functioning of the heart. The second, flat phase probably represents a stage at which production of ATP by augmented anaerobic glycolysis just balanced with the decreased utilization of this substance attributable to a stoppage of contractile activity. The third phase—a gradual decline—possibly

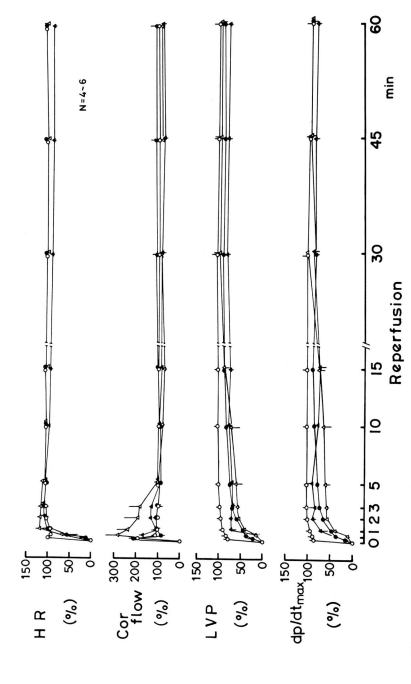

FIG. 13. Effects of reperfusion after occlusion of coronary inflow on the mechanical performances of the isolated perfused heart preparation. Values are expressed as percentage of the preocclusion values. Abbreviations are given in Fig. 1 and symbols are given in Fig. 8.

represents a stage at which the anerobic glycolysis failed to cope with even the low energy requirement of quiescent cells because of a depression of glycolysis. Depression of glycolysis is reported to be a characteristic feature of long-lasting ischemia (18,21).

With occlusions of longer than 1 min no restitution of ATP was observed even after 1 hr of reperfusion, whereas the myocardial creatine phosphate content was restored to a certain extent. A postanoxic failure of the myocardium to reaccumulate ATP has already been noted (2,5), although the cause and significance of this failure are not entirely clear. Benson et al. (2) considered it to be related in some way to the degradation of adenine nucleotides by deamination to hypoxanthine nucleotides. It is well established that oxygen deficiency causes an increased formation of ammonia in cardiac tissue owing to the deamination of AMP and adenosine (4,6). Regeneration of adenine nucleotides from hypoxanthine nucleotides took place, not by reversal of the degradation process, but by other mechanisms requiring oxygen and occurring relatively slowly. An alternate way of supplementing the loss of adenine nucleotides from the heart—the *de novo* synthesis—has also been shown to proceed rather slowly (22). Furthermore, deaminated nucleosides and bases leak out of the cell, thus producing a loss of substrate at intracellular sites where regeneration of nucleotides takes place.

In the present study, no correlation was observed between the myocardial content of ATP and the mechanical performances of the heart. During the period of ischemia, the contractile activity ceased at a time when half the initial value of ATP was still present, and the mechanical performances of the heart were quite well restored upon reperfusion, although there was no definite restitution of ATP. Furthermore, the myocardial ATP content was lower at certain times during the recovery process from ischemia than at the peak of ischemic insults. These findings indicate that the myocardial content of ATP does not necessarily represent the energy status of the myocardium, which must have been in a good state soon after the resumption of perfusion, since the mechanical performances of the heart were quite well reversed and the lactate accumulation was no longer observed at that time.

Although the myocardial content of creatine phosphate and the secondary parameters calculated from the values of adenine nucleotides and P_i seem to be correlated to the restitution process of the mechanical performances of the heart to a certain degree, further experiments are needed to draw any definite conclusion.

The amount of lactate accumulated within the myocardium during the ischemic period paralleled the duration of occlusion, if the duration of the ischemic period was not too long, thereby indicating that lactate content may be used as an alternate index of the severity of metabolic derangement produced by ischemic insult. The fact that accumulation of lactate tended to level off with longer ischemia is in agreement with the reports of previous workers that showed that the augmentation of glycolysis could not be maintained in the ischemic myocardium as opposed to that in the hypoxic myocardium (18,21).

The amount of lactate released into the perfusate upon reperfusion paralleled the amount accumulated during the ischemic period, which suggests that the lactate output from the heart could conveniently be used as a measure of the severity of metabolic derangement produced by ischemic insult.

REFERENCES

1. Atkinson, D. E., and Walton, G. M. (1967): Adenosine triphosphate conservation in metabolic regulation. Rat liver citrate cleavage enzyme. *J. Biol. Chem.,* 242:3239–3241.
2. Benson, E. S., Evans, G. T., Hallaway, B. E., Phibbs, C., and Freier, E. F. (1961): Myocardial creatine phosphate and nucleotides in anoxic cardiac arrest and recovery. *Am. J. Physiol.,* 201:687–693.
3. Bing, O. H. L., Apstein, C. S., and Brooks, W. W. (1975): Factors influencing tolerance of cardiac muscle to hypoxia. In: *Recent Advances in Studies on Cardiac Structure and Metabolism. Volume 10,* pp. 343–354. University Park Press, Baltimore.
4. Burger, R., and Lowenstein, J. M. (1967): Adenylate deaminase. III. Regulation of deamination pathways in extracts of rat heart and lung. *J. Biol. Chem.,* 242:5281–5288.
5. Coffman, J. D., Lewis, F. B., and Gregg, D. E. (1960): Effects of prolonged periods of anoxia on atrioventricular conduction and cardiac muscle. *Circ. Res.,* 8:649–659.
6. Deuticke, B., and Gerlach, E. (1966): Abbau freier Nucleotide in Herz, Skeletmuskel, Gehirn und Leber der Ratte bei Sauerstoffmangel. *Pfluegers Arch.,* 292:239–254.
7. Fawaz, G., and Fawaz, E. N. (1971): Phosphate compound analyses. In: *Methods in Pharmacology. Volume 1,* edited by A. Schwartz, pp. 515–551. Appleton-Century-Crofts, New York.
8. Feinstein, M. B. (1962): Effects of experimental congestive heart failure, ouabain, and asphyxia on the high-energy phosphate and creatine content of the guinea pig heart. *Circ. Res.,* 10:333–346.
9. Fiske, C. H., and Subbarow, Y. (1925): The colorimetric determination of phosphorus. *J. Biol. Chem.,* 66:375–400.
10. Furnival, C. M., Linden, R. J., and Snow, H. M. (1970): Inotropic changes in the left ventricle: The effect of changes in heart rate, aortic pressure and end-diastolic pressure. *J. Physiol.,* 211:359–387.
11. Gudbjarnason, S., Hayden, R. O., Wendt, V. E., Stock, T. B., and Bing, R. J. (1962): Oxidation reduction in heart muscle. Theoretical and clinical considerations. *Circulation,* 26:937–945.
12. Gudbjarnason, S., Mathes, P., and Ravens, K. G. (1970): Functional compartmentation of ATP and creatine phosphate in heart muscle. *J. Mol. Cell. Cardiol.,* 1:325–339.
13. Imai, S., Riley, A. L., and Berne, R. M. (1964): Effects of ischemia on adenine nucleotides in cardiac and skeletal muscle. *Circ. Res.,* 15:443–450.
14. Jones, C. E., Parker, J. C., and Smith, E. E. (1972): Determination of myocardial acid-soluble adenine nucleotides on anion-exchange thin layers. *J. Chromatogr.,* 64:378–382.
15. Kübler, W., and Spieckermann, P. G. (1970): Regulation of glycolysis in the ischemic and the anoxic myocardium. *J. Mol. Cell. Cardiol.,* 1:351–377.
16. Lehninger, A. L. (1975): *Biochemistry.* Worth Publishers, New York.
17. Maroko, P. R., Kjekshus, J. K., Sobel, B. E., Watanabe, T., Covell, J. W., Ross, J. K., Jr., and Braunwald, E. (1971): Factors influencing infarct size following experimental coronary artery occlusions. *Circulation,* 43:67–82.
18. Neely, J. R., Rovetto, M. J., Whitmer, J. T., and Morgan, H. E. (1973): Effects of ischemia on function and metabolism of the isolated working rat heart. *Am. J. Physiol.,* 225:651–658.
19. Otorii, T., Takeda, K., Katano, Y., Nakagawa, Y., and Imai, S. (1977): Effects of catecholamines on the myocardial redox potential. *Jpn. J. Pharmacol.,* 27:553–562.
20. Passonneau, J. V., and Lowry, O. H. (1974): Pyruvate. Fluorimetric assay. In: *Methods of Enzymatic Analysis. Volume 3,* edited by H. U. Bergmeyer, pp. 1452–1456. Academic Press, New York.
21. Rovetto, M. J., Whitmer, J. T., and Neely, J. R. (1973): Comparison of the effects of anoxia and whole heart ischemia on carbohydrate utilization in isolated, working rat heart. *Circ. Res.,* 32:699–711.
22. Zimmer, H.-Z., Trendelenburg, C., Kammermeier, H., and Gerlach, E. (1973): De novo synthesis of myocardial adenine nucleotides in the rat. Acceleration during recovery from oxygen deficiency. *Circ. Res.,* 32:635–642.

Ischemic Myocardium and Antianginal Drugs,
edited by M. M. Winbury and Y. Abiko.
Raven Press, New York © 1979.

Cyclic AMP and Arrhythmias

L. H. Opie and *W. F. Lubbe

*MRC Ischaemic Heart Disease Research Unit, Department of Medicine, Groote Schuur
Hospital, and University of Cape Town Medical School,
7925 Cape Town, South Africa*

A hypothesis has been proposed (14) linking accumulation of tissue cyclic
AMP to the development of ventricular fibrillation in the early period of developing myocardial infarction (11–13). This article briefly reviews the evidence for
that hypothesis.

BABOON DATA

The initial and fundamental observation, made in collaboration with Podzuweit et al. (13), was that after ligation of the coronary arteries in the baboon,
usually 25 to 30 min later, ventricular fibrillation developed. These were low-
level left anterior descending ligations and even though the infarct size was
small, the incidence of ventricular fibrillation was high. Baboons were more
susceptible to ventricular fibrillation than dogs, and the critical factor might
be that the tissue cyclic AMP in the ischemic zone increased in baboons, but
not to the same extent in dogs. A similar increase in the tissue cyclic AMP,
coinciding with the development of malignant arrhythmias, has been found in
the cat heart by Corr et al. (1). In our experimental conditions, the cyclic
AMP level in the normal ischemic zone stayed constant after ligation in both
baboons and dogs. Whether changes are present or not present in the nonischemic
zone is probably related to the size of the ischemic zone and the degree of
sympathetic stimulation; the latter factor would explain the rise of cyclic AMP
in both ischemic and nonischemic zones found by Wollenberger's group [Krause·
et al. (5)].

It should be noted that the cause of the rise of tissue cyclic AMP in the
baboon model is not known. There may be increased adenyl cyclase activity,
and the rat heart data suggest that β blockade should be effective in preventing
a ligation-induced rise of tissue cyclic AMP (Lubbe et al., *unpublished data*).
But data from the cat heart (1) and the pig heart (11) (C. A. Muller, L. H.
Opie, and W. F. Lubbe, *in preparation*) suggest that β blockade is only partially
effective in decreasing cyclic AMP in the ischemic zone. Other factors may

---

* Present address: Green Lane Hospital, Green Lane West, Auckland 3, New Zealand.

be at work, such as inhibition of phosphodiesterase activity by an increasingly low pH. Alternatively, adenyl cyclase activity may be stimulated by β-adrenergic drive but decreased by another temporary event, such as adenosine release; cessation of adenosine production could then, hypothetically, allow increased adenyl cyclase activity.

VENTRICULAR FIBRILLATION THRESHOLD

Is the association between cyclic AMP and arrhythmias a coincidence? Theoretically, β-adrenergic stimulation could be acting by another mechanism not involving cyclic AMP, with a coincidental rise in cyclic AMP. To show a direct causal relationship between cyclic AMP and ventricular fibrillation, an isolated perfused rat heart model was used to study the vulnerable period (7,9,10). By first giving a single stimulus, it was possible to define the currents in milliamps required to produce ventricular fibrillation at a given time in the cardiac cycle. By then giving a train of stimuli, it was possible to define the duration of the vulnerable period. Thus, the vulnerable period was defined in two dimensions (i.e., time and current) thereby defining a *multicornered vulnerable area*, the base of which was the duration of the vulnerable period and the apex of which was the ventricular fibrillation threshold (Fig. 1). The addition of epinephrine

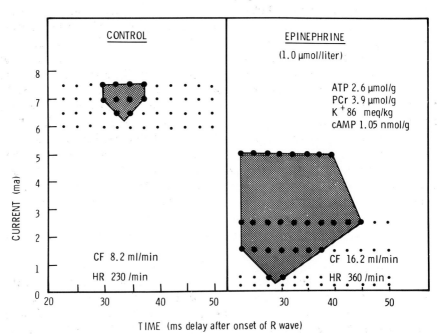

FIG. 1. Multicornered vulnerable area *(hatch-marked area)* in control rat heart in contrast to vulnerable area in epinephrine-treated rat heart (epinephrine = 10^{-6} M). Note widening of the vulnerable period (base of vulnerable zone), decrease of ventricular fibrillation threshold (minimum current required at apex of vulnerable zone), and overall increase of vulnerable area. For explanation of metabolic data, see Lubbe et al. (9). CF, coronary flow; HR, heart rate; PCr, phosphocreatine. (From Opie and Lubbe, ref. 10, with permission.)

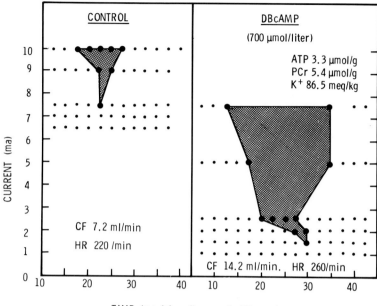

FIG. 2. Multicornered vulnerable area *(hatch-marked area)* in rat heart perfused with added dibutyryl cyclic AMP. Note marked widening of vulnerable period (base of vulnerable area), decrease of ventricular fibrillation threshold, and overall increase in vulnerable area (i.e., similar effects to those of epinephrine). For explanation of metabolic data, see Lubbe et al. (10). CF, coronary flow; HR, heart rate; PCr, phosphocreatine; DB cAMP, dibutyryl cyclic adenosine monophosphate. (From Opie and Lubbe, ref. 10, with permission.)

(10^{-6} M) caused a widening of the vulnerable period and a marked decrease in the current required to produce ventricular fibrillation (i.e., a fall in the ventricular fibrillation threshold), with an overall enlargement of the multicornered vulnerable area (Fig. 1). Tissue contents of ATP, phosphocreatine, and potassium underwent no consistent changes during epinephrine stimulation, but cyclic AMP doubled [See Table 1 of Lubbe et al. (9)]. Although epinephrine increased the heart rate, it was not the tachycardia that was responsible for the change in the multicornered vulnerable area because pacing at 300 or 400 beats/min did not alter the fibrillation threshold from the control value of 7.5 ± 0.4 mA ($n = 75$) at a heart rate of 262 ± 4 beats/min.

To support the hypothesis that cyclic AMP itself was mediating the changes in the multicornered vulnerable area, the vulnerable period, and the ventricular fibrillation threshold, hearts were perfused with exogenous cyclic AMP (9) or exogenous dibutyryl cyclic AMP (Figs. 2 and 3). In hearts perfused with cyclic AMP, there were no changes of note in the multicornered vulnerable area, but in the presence of dibutyryl cyclic AMP, there was a dose–response relationship between the amount added and the change in the fibrillation thresh-

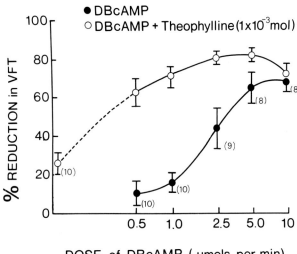

FIG. 3. Dose–response curves for effect of dibutyryl cyclic AMP (DB cAMP) in reducing the ventricular fibrillation threshold (VFT). Note that addition of theophylline greatly sensitizes the heart to low concentrations of dibutyryl cyclic AMP. Number of hearts studied are in parentheses.

old (Fig. 3). There was the theoretical possibility that dibutyryl cyclic AMP might have effects not only by penetrating the cell membrane but also by activating adenyl cyclase. The experiments were, therefore, repeated in the presence of atenolol, a cardiospecific β-1 blocking agent. The dose–response curve was unchanged in the presence of atenolol, which shows that adenyl cyclase activation was not involved and supports the alternate possibility that there was actual intracellular penetration of cyclic AMP in the dibutyryl form.

When theophylline was added to inhibit phosphodiesterase inhibition, there was a marked decrease in the fibrillation threshold for any given concentration of dibutyryl cyclic AMP (Fig. 3). Although externally added cyclic AMP had no effect on the fibrillation threshold, when it was added in the presence of theophylline, the fibrillation threshold fell (9). Thus, cyclic AMP itself might have slowly penetrated into the cell, to be broken down by phosphodiesterase; but when phosphodiesterase activity was inhibited by theophylline, then externally added cyclic AMP apparently could accumulate within the cell to change the ventricular fibrillation threshold.

But none of the above data actually proved that there was a direct relationship between the intracellular content of cyclic AMP and the fibrillation threshold in this model. The firmest data concerned the relationship between tissue cyclic AMP and the ventricular fibrillation threshold during the effects of β-1 stimulation obtained by comparing the effects of epinephrine, epinephrine plus atenolol, and epinephrine plus theophylline. During these procedures, tissue ATP was unchanged and tissue phosphocreatine, if anything, rose rather than fell (Fig.

4). Thus, we were not dealing with the sort of effects described by Fleckenstein, where epinephrine caused a marked decrease in the myocardial content of high-energy phosphates (3). As the epinephrine concentration in the rat heart perfusate increased, the fibrillation threshold fell and tissue cyclic AMP rose (Fig. 4).

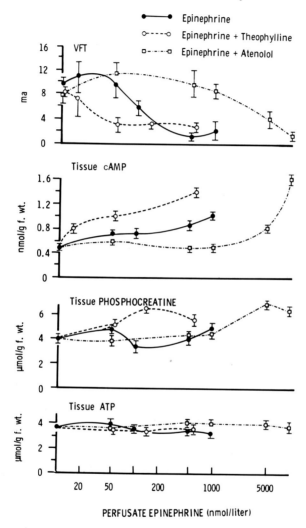

FIG. 4. Effect of increasing perfusate epinephrine concentrations on ventricular fibrillation threshold (VFT) (in milliamps), tissue cyclic AMP, tissue phosphocreatine, and tissue ATP in isolated perfused rat heart. Note that, as the tissue perfusate epinephrine increases, the ventricular fibrillation threshold falls and the cyclic AMP rises. Changes in high-energy phosphates are not consistent. In the presence of theophylline, tissue cyclic AMP rises much more markedly for any given epinephrine concentration, and the ventricular fibrillation threshold falls more rapidly. In the presence of β-1 cardiospecific blocker atenolol, the rise in tissue cyclic AMP is much delayed, as is the fall in the ventricular fibrillation threshold. (From Lubbe et al., ref. 9; reproduced by courtesy of the *Journal of Clinical Investigation*.)

In the presence of β-1 inhibition by atenolol, the curve for the fibrillation threshold shifted markedly to the right. The curve for cyclic AMP also shifted in a very similar way to the right, and there was a good relationship between the increase in the tissue cyclic AMP and the decrease in the ventricular fibrillation threshold in the various conditions studied. When the tissue cyclic AMP content for any given epinephrine concentration was increased by the addition of theophylline, the fibrillation threshold fell as the tissue cyclic AMP rose (Fig. 4). Therefore, it was reasonable of Lubbe et al. (7,9,10) to postulate that changes in the intracellular levels of cyclic AMP were mediating the changes in the fibrillation threshold.

SPONTANEOUS ARRHYTHMIAS AFTER CORONARY LIGATION

A criticism of the above data is that they relate to the effects of cyclic AMP on the ventricular fibrillation threshold, which may not necessarily be the same as having an effect on ischemic arrhythmias. To counter that criticism, Didier and Opie (2) evolved a system for quantifying arrhythmias after coronary artery ligation in the isolated rat heart. Isolated perfused rat hearts were subjected to coronary artery ligation by the method of Kannengiesser et al. (4) and continuous traces were made of the electrocardiogram. In hearts that were perfused with glucose, only occasional ventricular premature systoles developed (Fig. 5), and rather infrequently there was the development of periods of ventricular tachycardia or fibrillation.

Quantification of the arrhythmias was achieved by counting the number of

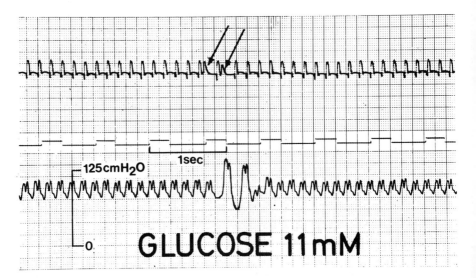

FIG. 5. Low incidence of ventricular premature systoles in coronary-ligated rat heart perfused with glucose (11 mM). For details of model, see Kannengiesser et al. (4).

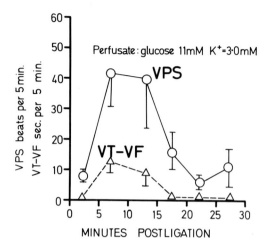

FIG. 6. Pattern of occurrence of ventricular premature systoles (VPS) *(open circles)* and ventricular tachycardia (VT) and/or ventricular fibrillation (VF) *(open triangles)* after coronary artery ligation of isolated perfused rat heart. For method of quantification of arrhythmias, see Didier and Opie (2). Note major incidence of arrhythmias in first 15 min postligation.

ventricular premature systoles in each 5-min period of perfusion after coronary ligation, and the duration of ventricular tachycardia or fibrillation per 5-min period was measured and quantified as the number of seconds of such an arrhythmia per 5-min period (Fig. 6). It is recognized that, owing to imperfections in the electrocardiogram, supraventricular tachycardias may have been included with the ventricular tachycardia–ventricular fibrillation classification.

With the addition of dibutyryl cyclic AMP, there was a greatly increased incidence of ventricular tachycardia and fibrillation (Fig. 7). The addition of epinephrine also increased the incidence of ventricular tachycardia and fibrillation, as well as the number of ventricular premature systoles (Tables 1 and 2). Coronary artery ligation itself had a major arrhythmogenic effect (8), and we (10) have also shown that coronary ligation increases tissue cyclic AMP and decreases the fibrillation threshold in the isolated nonworking rat heart model. It seemed reasonable, therefore, to anticipate that the same agents (coronary ligation and epinephrine) would increase tissue cyclic AMP in the ischemic zone in this isolated working rat heart model (Table 3).

Enzyme release from the coronary-ligated rat heart was also increased by agents that elevated cyclic AMP (ligation, ligation plus adrenaline, and, presumably, ligation plus dibutyryl cyclic AMP), which could, therefore, have increased the incidence of arrhythmias by increasing the severity of ischemic damage (Table 4). Thus, in this model we could not exclude a further complexity, namely, that cyclic AMP-mediated arrythmias were caused by an increase in the extent of ischemic damage as indicated by increased enzyme release. The alternate possibility, that the arrhythmias caused enzyme release by virtue of the arrhythmia-induced drop of arterial perfusion pressure, was unlikely because the diastolic arterial perfusion pressure, largely responsible for coronary artery perfusion, was unchanged (the perfusion pressure was maintained by the apparatus; see Fig. 7). Horak and Opie have suggested that cyclic AMP may in some way

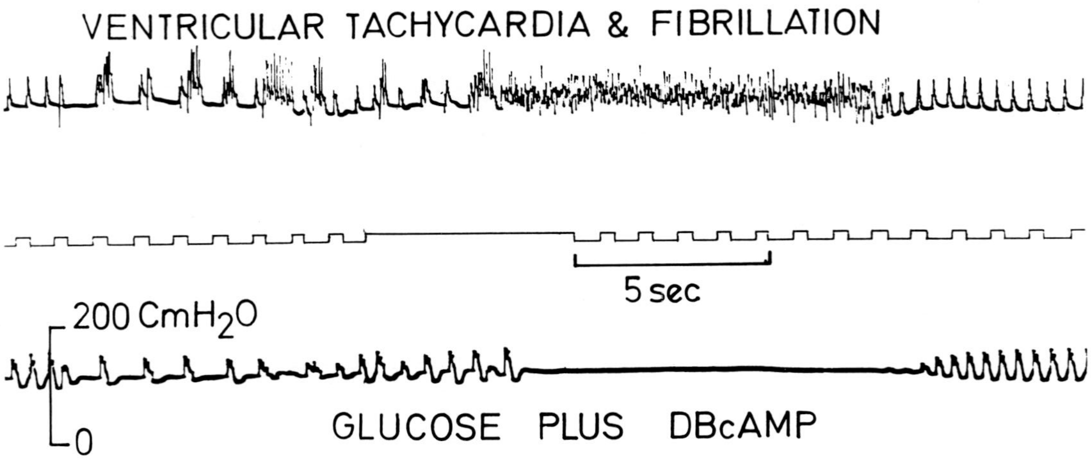

FIG. 7. Effect of addition of dibutyryl cyclic AMP (DB cAMP, 5 mM) on spontaneous arrhythmias after coronary artery ligation in rat heart. Note the runs of ventricular tachycardia and fibrillation and the loss of aortic pressure with these arrhythmias.

TABLE 1. *Postligation ventricular premature systoles (VPS) and effect of agents thought to elevate tissue cyclic AMP in isolated working rat heart*

Condition	VPS[a] (beats per 5 min)	p (vs glucose)
Glucose (11 mM)	20.9 ± 3.9 (n = 96)	
Glucose + dibutyryl cyclic AMP (5 mM)	77.0 ± 11.3 (n = 52)	< 0.001
Glucose + epinephrine (10^{-7} M)	55.3 ± 13.2 (n = 32)	< 0.02

[a] Mean values ± SEM. n = Number of 5-min periods studied (see Fig. 6).

TABLE 2. *Postligation ventricular tachycardia–ventricular fibrillation (VT–VF) and agents thought to elevate tissue cyclic AMP in isolated perfused working rat heart*

Condition	VT–VF[a] (sec per 5 min)	p (vs glucose)
Glucose 11 mM	5.1 ± 1.4 (n = 96)	
Glucose + dibutyryl cyclic AMP (5 mM)	42.3 ± 10.1 (n = 52)	< 0.001
Glucose + epinephrine (10^{-7} M)	62.2 ± 17.4 (n = 36)	< 0.003

[a] n = Number of 5-min periods studied (see Fig. 6).

TABLE 3. *Tissue cyclic AMP in ischemic zone of coronary-ligated isolated working heart*

	Cyclic AMP content[a] (nmoles/g wet wt)	p (vs control)
Preligation	0.48 ± 0.03 (n = 8)	
Ligation (10 min)[b]	0.65 ± 0.04 (n = 4)	< 0.01
Ligation + epinephrine (10 min)	0.86 ± 0.09 (n = 6)	< 0.01

[a] n = Number of hearts studied.
[b] These are preliminary observations; note the small numbers.

increase membrane permeability and thereby hasten enzyme release (A. Horak and L. H. Opie, *in preparation*).

HYPOTHETICAL EFFECTS OF CYCLIC AMP

Cyclic AMP may have at least four ways of producing ventricular arrhythmias: (a) Cyclic AMP may cause calcium-dependent slow responses (Fig. 8) that occur especially in potassium-blocked fibers (12); although this mechanism

TABLE 4. *Postligation release of lactate dehydrogenase (LDH) and effect of agents thought to elevate tissue cyclic AMP in isolated working rat heart*

Condition	Release of LDH[a] (mU/g/min)	p (vs glucose alone)
Glucose	95 ± 8 ($n = 48$)	
Glucose + dibutyryl cyclic AMP (5 mM)	232 ± 31 ($n = 23$)	< 0.001
Glucose + epinephrine (10^{-7} M)	374 ± 50 ($n = 15$)	< 0.0001

[a]n = Number of 5-min periods studied (see Fig. 6).

should be sensitive to calcium-blocking agents, verapamil did not inhibit postligation ventricular arrhythmias in our pig model (C. A. Muller, L. H. Opie, and W. F. Lubbe, *in preparation*). (b) Cyclic AMP may cause afterpotentials (6). (c) Cyclic AMP may also cause increased automaticity in Purkinje fibers (16). (d) Theoretically, cyclic AMP may be instrumental in the accumulation of complex phospholipids that cause multiple electrophysiological abnormalities (15). The latter possibility is an extension of the postulated relation between cyclic AMP and lipolysis in the ischemic myocardium (Fig. 8).

The hypothesis relating cyclic AMP to the occurrence of ventricular arrhyth-

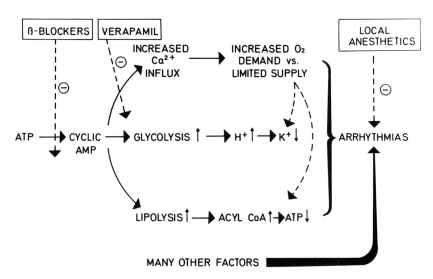

FIG. 8. Original hypothesis on proposed relationship between cyclic AMP and development of ventricular arrhythmias. [see Podzuweit et al. (14)]. The original hypothesis stressed (a) the effect of cyclic AMP in promotion of Ca^{2+} entry into the heart, thereby increasing the metabolic gradients between ischemic and nonischemic tissue; (b) the metabolic effects of cyclic AMP on glycogenolysis and lipolysis; and (c) the electrophysiological effects of cyclic AMP. (From Podzuweit et al., ref. 14, by permission of the Editors, *Lancet.*)

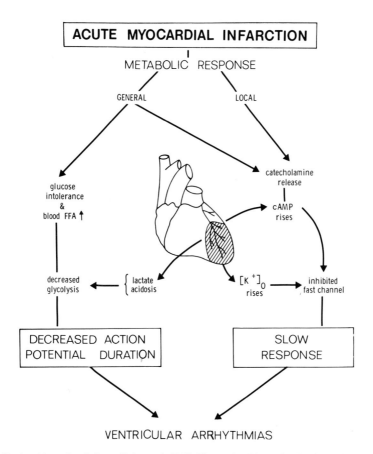

ACUTE MYOCARDIAL INFARCTION

METABOLIC RESPONSE

GENERAL   LOCAL

glucose
intolerance
&
blood FFA ↑

catecholamine
release

cAMP
rises

decreased
glycolysis

lactate
acidosis

$[K^+]_0$
rises

inhibited
fast channel

DECREASED ACTION
POTENTIAL DURATION

SLOW
RESPONSE

VENTRICULAR ARRHYTHMIAS

FIG. 9. Revised hypothesis [see Opie et al. (11)]. The revised hypothesis allows for a complex genesis of ventricular arrhythmias in acute myocardial infarction [see also Opie et al. (12)]. Two of the possible mechanisms are shown in this scheme. First, an elevation of cyclic AMP in the ischemic zone could, in the presence of increased external potassium, provoke the slow response. Second, a decreased action potential duration has been linked to conditions decreasing glycolysis, such as accumulation of lactate and protons. These local metabolic changes may be related to the general metabolic response, which includes catecholamine release, glucose intolerance, and increased blood free fatty acids. For further details, see Opie et al. (11). (From Opie, Muller, and Lubbe, ref. 11, by permission of the Editors, *Lancet.*)

mias is subject to a number of criticisms (12), including the following. First, cyclic AMP is likely to be only an initiator of a chain of further intracellular events, probably involving protein kinase activation. These further events are, at present, quite unknown. Second, it would be a gross and serious oversimplification to suppose that cyclic AMP is the only arrhythmogenic agent at work, especially in the very complex setting of regional ischemia (Fig. 9). Especially in patients, the combination of varying degrees of coronary artery disease, coronary spasm, past ischemia, and complex conduction disturbances may all play alternate or additional roles to cyclic AMP in producing arrhythmias. It would not be surprising if further work were to find situations in which cyclic AMP rises and ventricular fibrillation are not linked. Nevertheless, on present evidence, we suggest that cyclic AMP may reasonably be considered to be one of the important factors in the production of ischemic arrhythmias.

ACKNOWLEDGMENTS

We thank Dr. T. Podzuweit and Owen Bricknell, B.Sc., for collaborative work and useful discussions and the Medical Research Council and the Chris Barnard fund for support of the original work cited.

REFERENCES

1. Corr, P. B., Witkowski, F. X., and Sobel, B. E. (1978): Mechanisms contributing to malignant dysrhythmias induced by ischemia in the cat. *J. Clin. Invest.,* 61:109–119.
2. Didier, J. P., and Opie, L. H. (1979): Effect of glucose and fatty acids and of coronary ligation on isolated perfused working rat hearts. *J. Mol. Cell. Cardiol. (in press).*
3. Fleckenstein, A. (1971): Specific inhibitors and promoters of calcium action in the excitation-contraction coupling of heart muscle and their role in the prevention or production of myocardial lesions. In: *Calcium and the Heart,* edited by P. Harris and L. H. Opie, pp. 135–188. Academic Press, London.
4. Kannengiesser, G. J., Lubbe, W. F., and Opie, L. H. (1975): Experimental myocardial infarction with left ventricular failure in the isolated perfused rat heart: Effects of isoproterenol and pacing. *J. Mol. Cell. Cardiol.,* 7:135–151.
5. Krause, E.-G., Ziegelhöffer, A., Fedelvosa, M., Styk, J., Kostolanski, S., Gabauer, I., Blasig, I., and Wollenberger, A. (1978): Myocardial cyclic nucleotide levels following coronary artery ligation. *Adv. Cardiol.,* 25:119–129.
6. Lazzara, R., Hope, R. R., and Yeh, B. K. (1978): Implication of cAMP and calcium as mediators of automaticity induced in working myocardium. *Am. J. Cardiol.,* 41:417 (Abstract).
7. Lubbe, W. F., Bricknell, O. L., Podzuweit, T., and Opie, L. H. (1976): Cyclic AMP as a determinant of vulnerability to ventricular fibrillation. *Cardiovasc. Res.,* 10:697–702.
8. Lubbe, W. F., Daries, P., and Opie, L. H. (1978): Ventricular arrhythmias associated with coronary artery occlusion and reperfusion in the isolated perfused rat heart: A model for assessment of antifibrillatory action of antiarrhythmic agents. *Cardiovasc. Res.,* 12:212–220.
9. Lubbe, W. F., Podzuweit, T., Daries, P. S., and Opie, L. H. (1978): The role of cyclic adenosine monophosphate in adrenergic effects on vulnerability to fibrillation in the isolated perfused rat heart. *J. Clin. Invest.,* 6:1260–1269.
10. Opie, L. H., and Lubbe, W. F. (1979): Catecholamine-mediated arrhythmias in acute myocardial infarction: Experimental evidence and role of beta-blockade. *S. Afr. Med. J. (in press).*
11. Opie, L. H., Muller, C. A., and Lubbe, W. F. (1978): Cyclic AMP and arrhythmias revisited. *Lancet,* 2:921–923.
12. Opie, L. H., Nathan, D., and Lubbe, W. F. (1979): Biochemical aspects of arrhythmogenesis and ventricular fibrillation. *Am. J. Cardiol.,* 43:131–148.
13. Podzuweit, T., Dalby, A. J., Cherry, G. W., and Opie, L. H. (1978): Cyclic AMP levels in ischaemic and non-ischaemic myocardium following coronary artery ligation: Relation to ventricular fibrillation. *J. Mol. Cell. Cardiol.,* 10:81–94.
14. Podzuweit, T., Lubbe, W. F., and Opie, L. H. (1976): Cyclic adenosine monophosphate, ventricular fibrillation and antiarrhythmic drugs. *Lancet,* 1:341–342.
15. Sobel, B. E., Corr, P. B., Robison, A. K., Goldstein, R. A., Witkowski, F. X., and Klein, M. S. (1978): Accumulation of lysophosphoglycerides with arrhythmogenic properties in ischemic myocardium. *J. Clin. Invest.,* 62:546–553.
16. Tsien, R. W., Giles, W., and Greengard, P. (1972): Cyclic AMP mediates the effects of adrenaline on cardiac Purkinje fibres. *Nature New Biol.,* 240:181–183.

Ischemic Myocardium and Antianginal Drugs,
edited by M. M. Winbury and Y. Abiko.
Raven Press, New York © 1979.

Cardiac Lipids and Ischemic Tolerance

Sigmundur Gudbjarnason and Jonas Hallgrimsson

Science Institute, University of Iceland, 107 Reykjavik, Iceland

The purpose of this study is to examine cardiac lipids in relation to coronary artery disease in the human heart and sudden cardiac death. We have examined the content and composition of free and esterified fatty acids in human heart muscle and modified the composition of cardiac phospholipids (PL) in experimental animals.

The major part of fatty acids in heart muscle is present in phospholipids. The phospholipids play an important role in structure and function of membranes, and the composition of these phospholipids is continuously modified by external and internal factors, such as diet or hormones.

MODIFICATION OF THE FATTY ACID COMPOSITION OF CARDIAC PHOSPHOLIPIDS

Not only is dietary fat involved in hyperlipemia and atherosclerosis, but it may also cause extensive alterations in the composition of cardiac lipids and thereby influence membrane properties and kinetic properties of membrane-bound enzymes. The fatty acid composition of cardiac phospholipids is modified in rats by feeding a diet containing 10% cod liver oil (CLO) for 3 or 9 months (6). The results reflect the dynamic state of esterified fatty acids in heart muscle lipids. There is an extensive replacement of endogenous fatty acids by exogenous fatty acids, such as the replacement of linoleic acid (18:2n6) and arachidonic acid (20:4n6) by docosahexaenoic acid (22:6n3). These alterations were more pronounced after 3 months than after 9 months of feeding the CLO, which suggests an adaptation to this dietary lipid (Table 1).

The longer and more unsaturated 22:6n3 replaces about one-third of 18:2n6 in phospholipids. The replacement of only one-third of 18:2n6 by 22:6n3 is due to the selective modification of individual phospholipids. There is an extensive modification of the polyene fatty acid composition of phosphatidyl ethanolamine (PE) and phosphatidyl choline (PC), whereas cardiolipin, which contains about 70% 18:2n6, is not significantly altered by the CLO diet. The resistance of cardiolipin to modification in fatty acid composition by dietary lipids is of particular interest because cardiolipin is located in the inner mitochondrial membrane and is associated with mitochondrial energy metabolism.

213

TABLE 1. *Percentage fatty acid composition of dietary cod liver oil and heart muscle lipids in control animals and animals fed 10% cod liver oil[a]*

Fatty acid	Dietary cod liver oil	Phospholipids		
		Control ($n = 12$)	Cod liver oil, 3 months ($n = 4$)	Cod liver oil, 9 months ($n = 6$)
14:0	4.1			
16:0 al		1.8 ± 0.2	4.3 ± 0.2^c	1.4 ± 0.2^d
16:0	10.0	12.4 ± 0.2	9.2 ± 0.4^c	11.5 ± 0.3
16:1n7	9.3			
18:0	2.6	19.4 ± 0.4	14.9 ± 0.3^c	21.1 ± 0.7^d
18:1n9	22.0	8.3 ± 0.3	5.8 ± 0.2^c	8.6 ± 0.4
18:2n6	2.1	26.7 ± 0.9	20.1 ± 0.5^c	19.6 ± 1.0^c
18:3n3	0.6^b			
20:1n9	11.8			
20:4n6		15.4 ± 0.5	9.0 ± 0.3^c	10.8 ± 0.4^c
20:5n3	10.0	0.2 ± 0.1	3.3 ± 0.2^c	2.8 ± 0.2^c
22:1n11	8.0			
22:5n3	1.5	1.5 ± 0.1	1.6 ± 0.1	1.4 ± 0.1
22:6n3	10.0	12.1 ± 0.7	29.1 ± 0.8^c	$18.3 \pm 1.1^{c,d}$

[a] Mean values $\pm$ SE for animals fed cod liver oil for 3 or 9 months.
[b] 18:3n3 + 20:0.
[c] $p < 0.001$, difference between control and experimental groups.
[d] $p < 0.01$, difference between groups of animals fed cod liver oil for 3 months, respectively.

Other methods are available to modify the fatty acid composition of cardiac phospholipids, e.g., various forms of stress. Norepinephrine injected in increasing amounts (1 to 5 mg/kg for 15 days) led to a significant increase in 22:6n3 and a corresponding decrease in 18:2n6 without affecting other fatty acids (Table 2) (4). Similar changes may be induced by chronic administration of nicotine to animals fed a high-cholesterol diet (1%) and by various other forms of stress,

TABLE 2. *Percentage fatty acid composition of cardiac phospholipids in control animals and animals treated daily with increasing doses of norepinephrine (1–5 mg/kg) for up to 15 days*

Fatty acid	Control ($n = 12$)	Norepinephrine ($n = 4$)
16:0	12.4 ± 0.2	12.0 ± 0.1
18:0	19.4 ± 0.4	22.2 ± 0.1
18:1n9	8.3 ± 0.3	7.4 ± 0.2
18:2n6	26.7 ± 0.9	15.6 ± 0.4^a
20:4n6	15.4 ± 0.5	17.6 ± 0.3
22:5n3	1.5 ± 0.1	1.4 ± 0.1
22:6n3	12.1 ± 0.7	20.0 ± 0.2^a

[a] $p < 0.001$.

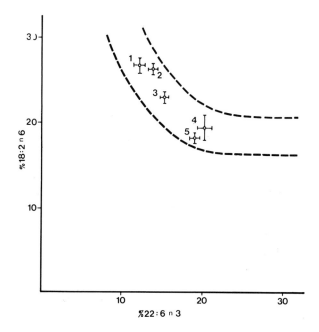

FIG. 1. The relationship between linoleic acid (18:2n6) and docosahexaenoic acid (22:6n3) in phospholipids of rat heart muscle. *1,* Control animals ($n = 12$). *2,* Rats fed a diet containing 1% cholesterol for 6 months ($n = 8$). *3,* Rats subjected to chronic administration of nicotine. Nicotine injected (0.5 mg/kg, s.c.) twice daily for 6 months ($n = 13$). *4,* Rats subjected to chronic administration of nicotine and fed a diet containing 1% cholesterol, as described above ($n = 8$). *5,* Rats injected with toxic doses of vitamin D_3 (3×10^5 U/day for 10 days) ($n = 4$).

such as toxic doses of vitamin D. In these various forms of stress there is an extensive replacement of 18:2n6 by 22:6n3 in specific phospholipids (Fig. 1).

CARDIAC LIPIDS AND CATECHOLAMINE TOLERANCE

What are the consequences of such changes in cardiac lipid composition? Do these changes affect ischemic tolerance or stress tolerance? We have examined the influence of dietary CLO on the development of cardiac necrosis and mortality following either isoproterenol stress or norepinephrine stress. These stress models may give some information on ischemic tolerance during excessive adrenergic stimulation. Isoproterenol causes hypotension and insufficient coronary perfusion, whereas norepinephrine does not cause ischemia. Excessive stimulation with both of these catecholamines results frequently in the development of cardiac necrosis and high mortality.

Isoproterenol was given according to the method of Rona: 40 mg/kg, injected twice, the second injection given 24 hr after the first. Following isoproterenol treatment, the control animals, which were fed a standard diet, had a mortality rate of 50%, whereas the animals that were fed a diet containing CLO had a mortality rate of 100%. When the rats were subjected to norepinephrine stress (1 to 5 mg/kg for 15 days), both control rats and rats fed the CLO diet had the same mortality rate, about 50%.

We are presently examining the possibility that the low isoproterenol tolerance of animals fed CLO may be due to impaired ischemic tolerance, which could be the result of altered membrane composition and stability.

POLYENE FATTY ACIDS AND CARDIOTOXICITY OF CATECHOLAMINES

The fatty acid composition of cardiac membrane lipids could influence the cardiotoxicity of catecholamines in several ways. There may be a direct relation-

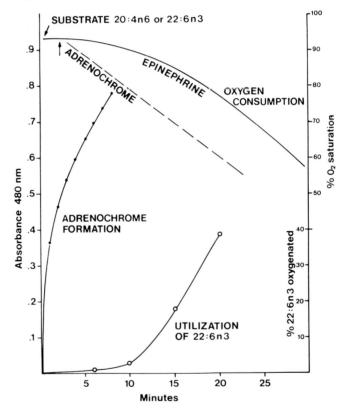

FIG. 2. Polyene fatty acid-stimulated adrenochrome formation and catecholamine-stimulated peroxidation of polyene fatty acids. Assay conditions: (a) Adrenochrome formation—22.3 μg protein, 1 mM epinephrine, 50 mM Tris pH 8.3, 8.33 mM sucrose, 0.66 mM 20:4n6 or 22:6n3. (b) Oxygenase activity—24 μg protein, 1 mM epinephrine, 50 mM Tris pH 8.3, 10.7 mM sucrose, 0.086 mM MgCl$_2$, 0.57 mM 20:4n6 or 22:6n3, final volume 3.5 ml. (c) Utilization of 22:6n3— 50 ml final volume, 9-ml aliquots for time points; 327 μg protein, 1 mM epinephrine, 50 mM Tris pH 8.3, 10.7 mM sucrose, 0.086 mM MgCl$_2$, 0.57 mM 22:6n3, analyses of 22:6n3 by gas–liquid chromatography.

ship between catecholamine and polyene fatty acid metabolism in the heart. Yates and Dhalla (8) have suggested that the cardiotoxicity of catecholamines is primarily due to the corresponding aminochrome (i.e., oxidation products of the catecholamine). They observed, in isolated rat hearts perfused with oxidized isoproterenol, ultrastructural changes and impairment of the functional capacity of cardiac muscle that led in a short time to complete failure of contractility.

Polyene fatty acids, both $20:4n6$ and $22:6n3$, stimulate microsomal oxidation of epinephrine to adrenochrome. The adrenochrome in turn stimulates microsomal peroxidation or oxygenation of the polyene fatty acids to various fatty acid derivatives. Figure 2 shows a time lag for the epinephrine-stimulated oxygen consumption (i.e., oxygenation and utilization of $22:6n3$). Replacement of epinephrine with adrenochrome eliminates this lag, which suggests that the oxidation product of epinephrine, (i.e., adrenochrome) stimulates the oxygenation of polyene fatty acids. This time lag is not observed for the polyene fatty acid-stimulated adrenochrome formation. This suggests that these reactions are catalyzed by two separate enzyme systems. These enzymes can be inhibited individually. Propranolol, for example, inhibits epinephrine oxidation to adrenochrome without inhibiting the adrenochrome-stimulated oxygenation of polyene fatty acids. Vitamin E inhibits the oxygenation of polyene fatty acids without inhibiting adrenochrome formation. Indomethacin inhibits both adrenochrome formation and polyene fatty acid oxygenation.

Adrenochrome could affect catecholamine tolerance in several ways, for example (a) stimulating peroxidation of membrane polyene fatty acids and causing membrane damage and ultrastructural changes; or (b) inhibiting catechol-*O*-methyl transferase (COMT) (3), thereby diminishing the inactivation of released catecholamines and thus amplifying the catecholamine effects.

FUNCTION OF POLYENE FATTY ACIDS

We have seen that various forms of stress are accompanied by changes in fatty acid composition of cardiac phospholipids (i.e., by an extensive replacement of $18:2n6$ by $22:6n3$ in specific phospholipids). What are the functions of these fatty acids? $18:2n6$ is the precursor of $20:4n6$, which serves as a substrate for synthesis of endoperoxides, prostaglandins, prostacyclin, and other regulatory substances. The function of $22:6n3$ is unknown. $22:6n3$ is present in relatively large amounts in excitable tissue—the brain (7) and the retina of the eye (1). $22:6n3$ is also present in cardiac PL, and it may have a role to play in cardiac function. There is an exponential increase in cardiac PL docosapolyene fatty acids ($22:5n3 + 22:6n3$) with heart rate (from a heart rate of 8 to 10/min in the fin whale to 624/min in the mouse—see Fig. 3). The relationship between heart rate and $22:6n3$ in PE in heart muscle (Fig. 4) suggests that $22:6n3$ might participate in the regulation of membrane permeability, possibly forming a cation-conducting transmembrane channel, conceivably a Na^+ channel.

It is tempting to speculate how $22:6n3$ could form cation-conducting trans-

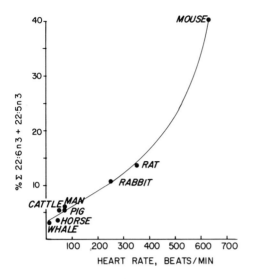

FIG. 3. Relationship between docosapolyene fatty acids (22:5n3 + 22:6n3) in cardiac phospholipids and heart rate of various mammals.

membrane channels. Conformational changes in 22:6n3 should accompany alterations in membrane structure and thickness induced by the membrane potential. Such thickness changes induced by the transmembrane potential have been demonstrated in black lipid membrane models by Benz and Janko (2). The voltage-induced capacitance changes or thickness changes are strongly dependent upon the lipid composition. The authors concluded from the small thickness of the compressed membranes (30 to 50 Å) that the hydrocarbon chains of the lipids must be more or less coiled. If similar thickness changes occur in the plasma membrane of the living cell, 22:6n3 could assume a spiral or helical form during a voltage-induced compression of the membrane, and two such

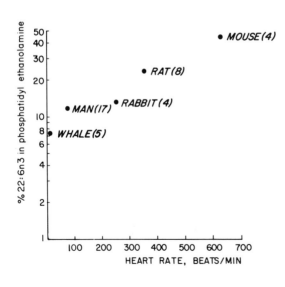

FIG. 4. Relationship between docosahexaenoic acid (22:6n3) in cardiac phosphatidyl ethanolamine and heart rate. Parentheses indicate number studied.

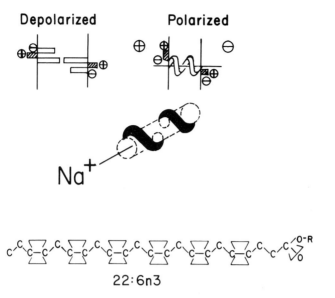

FIG. 5. Hypothetical comformational changes in phospholipid fatty acyl groups during a voltage-induced compression and thinning of the membrane. Two such opposite helical forms of 22:6n3 could form a cation-conducting channel.

opposing spirals or helixes could form a cation-conducting channel (Na^+ channel). This channel would be lined on the inside with π-electron orbitals liganding cations that are being transferred across the membrane. Each channel would possess 14 such π bonds facilitating the ion transfer. Depolarization and relaxation of the membrane increases membrane thickness, thereby inducing conformational changes in membrane-bound 22:6n3 from the spiral to a more stretched form when the transmembrane channel becomes closed and nonconducting (Fig. 5).

In this manner, 22:6n3 could participate in excitation. The rhythmic instability, which is characteristic of excitable tissue, would be caused by physical changes in the membrane as a result of physical forces, such as the electrochemical potential, fixed charges, and osmotic gradients. It should be noted that the ionic movements associated with excitation take place independently of those involved in active ion transport. The ionic movements that take place during depolarization are from areas (zones) of higher to those of lower concentration gradients. They require no energy and involve considerably greater fluxes than do active transport processes.

STUDIES ON HUMAN HEART MUSCLE

Studies on human cardiac autopsy samples suggest that changes in tissue levels of polyunsaturated fatty acids in myocardial phospholipids may be associated with coronary heart disease. Heart muscle samples were obtained from accident victims, and if these hearts were, on macroscopic and microscopic examination, without any lesions or abnormalities, they were considered normal. Samples were also obtained from heart muscle of people who died a sudden cardiac death, with or without coronary atherosclerosis. Sudden cardiac death is defined as instant death or death within 1 hr, usually within minutes, from symptoms of myocardial infarction (5).

Analyses of human autopsy material must be viewed with caution because of the autolytic changes that take place from the time of death until the time of sampling, often 20 to 36 hr. The autolytic changes in heart muscle are relatively slow compared to those in many other tissues, such as the liver.

First, we attempted to examine postmortem changes in cardiac lipids. There was no relationship between time of sampling after death and the amount of phospholipids or free fatty acids in the heart muscle samples. This could mean that the dynamic or metabolically more active phospholipids had already broken down before we obtained our earliest samples several hours after death.

Stability of Cardiac Phospholipids

The composition of free fatty acids (FFA) found in autopsy samples indicates that these FFA are primarily derived from hydrolysis of cardiac phospholipids.

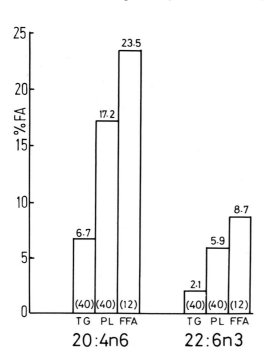

FIG. 6. Relative amounts of 20:4n6 and 22:6n3 in neutral lipids (TG), PL, and FFA in human cardiac muscle (autopsy). *Parentheses* indicate number studied.

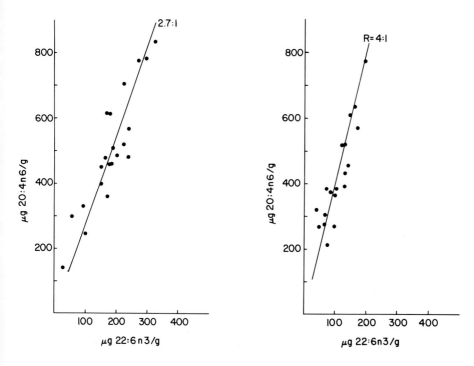

FIG. 7. Relationship between 20:4n6 and 22:6n3 in phosphatidyl ethanolamine **(left)** and phosphatidyl choline **(right)** in human heart muscle.

There is an important difference in composition of PL and FFA: The FFA contain relatively more of the polyene fatty acids 20:4n6 and 22:6n3 than found in remaining phospholipids (Fig. 6). This could mean that PL containing these fatty acids are more readily hydrolyzed by myocardial phospholipases than PL containing more saturated fatty acids. There also appears to be a faster breakdown of PL containing 22:6n3 than of PL containing 20:4n6.

There is a relationship between 20:4n6 and 22:6n3 in cardiac PE and PC (Fig. 7). The ratio of 20:4 to 22:6 is lower in PE than PC because 22:6n3 is present in relatively larger quantities in PE. This ratio is not constant; it decreases with age owing to an increase in 22:6n3 with age. The relationship between these two fatty acids in myocardial FFA, mostly released from the PL, shows that there is relatively more 22:6n3 in the FFA fraction than in PL, which suggests that PL containing 22:6n3 break down more readily than other PL (Fig. 8).

Individuals with myocardial infarction have a lower ratio of 20:3 to 22:6 in FFA than individuals with normal muscle, which indicates a greater breakdown of PE or PL containing 22:6n3 in the infarcted hearts.

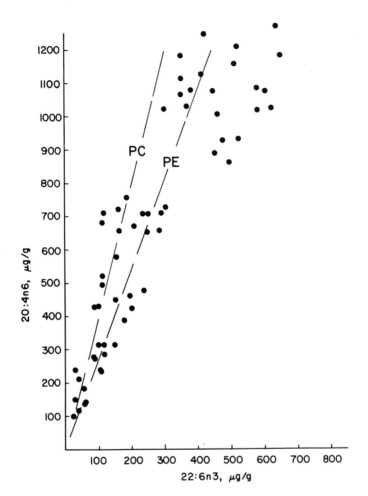

FIG. 8. Relationship between 20:4n6 and 22:6n3 in the FFA fraction of human heart muscle. PC and PE represent the myocardial phospholipids illustrated in Fig. 7.

Our observations suggest that the stability of cardiac phospholipids or the resistance to hydrolysis is a function of the fatty acid composition. The most unsaturated PL are the most unstable, and stability increases with the saturation of the fatty acids.

Myocardial Lipids and Coronary Atherosclerosis

In individuals with severe coronary atherosclerosis and coronary artery stenosis (grades 5 or 6), the following alterations in the cardiac lipids were observed:
(a) Cardiac phospholipids of normal muscle with severe coronary atherosclero-

sis showed a lower content of 18:2n6 compared to normal muscle with mild or no coronary atherosclerosis. This resembles stress adaptation in experimental animals.

(b) Cardiac glycerides are frequently increased in quantity in atherosclerotic hearts. The unsaturation of glyceride fatty acid increases with the glyceride content of the muscle, which suggests that the pathological glycerides may be derived from phospholipids by action of phospholipase C in an ischemic or energy-deficient muscle.

(c) The FFA levels of cardiac muscle are significantly lower in severely atherosclerotic hearts compared to mild or moderate atherosclerosis of accident victims.

Myocardial Lipids and Sudden Cardiac Death

In sudden cardiac death with mild or no coronary atherosclerosis, the following observations were made: (a) very high myocardial levels of FFA (14.2 ± 2.3 mg/g) derived from glycerides, normal phospholipids, no myocardial infarction; (b) elevated myocardial levels of FFA (6.2 ± 0.2 mg/g) derived from phospholipids and glycerides, low myocardial levels of PE and very low levels of 22:6n3, no myocardial infarction; (c) normal levels of myocardial FFA (4.3 ± 0.3 mg/g), abnormal glyceride composition, no myocardial infarction.

In sudden cardiac death with marked coronary artery stenosis (grades 5 or 6), the following observations were made: (a) very low levels of FFA (1.8 ± 0.5 mg/g); (b) frequent high levels of cardiac glycerides of abnormal composition; (c) frequent myocardial infarction.

These observations indicate that significant alterations in cardiac lipid metabolism are associated with coronary artery disease and with many cases of sudden cardiac death in the absence of coronary artery stenosis or myocardial infarction. Sudden cardiac death may be associated with membrane dysfunction due to breakdown of specific membrane lipids or membrane destabilization due to excessive cellular levels of FFA.

SUMMARY

The fatty acid composition of cardiac PL is modified by diet and stress. The catecholamine tolerance may be influenced by the composition of cardiac lipids. Polyene fatty acids stimulate oxidation of catecholamines to cardiotoxic aminochromes, which in turn accelerate peroxidation of polyene fatty acids. There is a relationship between heart rate and the docosahexaenoic acid, (22:6n3) content of cardiac phospholipids. Stability of cardiac phospholipids is a function of the fatty acid composition; the stability decreases with increasing unsaturation of fatty acids.

Alterations in human cardiac lipids are associated with (a) coronary atherosclerosis and (b) many cases of sudden cardiac death in the absence of marked coronary artery stenosis or myocardial infarction.

REFERENCES

1. Anderson, R. E. (1970): Lipids of ocular tissues. IV. A comparison of the phospholipids from the retina of six mammalian species. *Exp. Eye Res.,* 10:339–344.
2. Benz, R., and Janko, K. (1976): Voltage-induced capacitance relaxation of lipid bilayer membranes. Effects of membrane composition. *Biochim. Biophys. Acta,* 445:721–738.
3. Borchardt, T. R. (1975): Catechol-*O*-methyltransferase: A model to study the mechanism of 6-hydroxydopamine interaction with proteins. In *Chemical Tools in Catecholamine Research. Volume 1,* edited by G. Jonsson, T. Malmfors, and E. Sachs, pp. 33–40. North-Holland, Amsterdam.
4. Gudbjarnason, S., Doell, B., Óskarsdóttir, G., and Hallgrimsson, J. (1978): Modification of cardiac phospholipids and catecholamine stress tolerance. In *Tocopherol, Oxygen and Biomembranes,* edited by C. de Duve and O. Hayaishi, pp. 297–310. Elsevier/North-Holland, Amsterdam.
5. Gudbjarnason, S., and Hallgrimsson, J. (1975): The role of myocardial membrane lipids in the development of cardiac necrosis. *Acta Med. Scand. (Suppl.),* 587:17–26.
6. Gudbjarnason, S., and Óskarsdóttir, G. (1977): Modification of fatty acid composition of rat heart lipids by feeding cod liver oil. *Biochim. Biophys. Acta,* 487:10–15.
7. Svennerholm, L. (1968): Distribution and fatty acid composition of phosphoglycerides in normal human brain. *J. Lipid Res.,* 9:570–579.
8. Yates, J. C., and Dhalla, N. S. (1975): Induction of necrosis and failure in the isolated perfused rat heart with oxidized isoproterenol. *J. Mol. Cell. Cardiol.,* 7:807–816.

Ischemic Myocardium and Antianginal Drugs,
edited by M. M. Winbury and Y. Abiko.
Raven Press, New York © 1979.

Relationship Between Ventricular Function and Intermediates of Fatty Acid Metabolism During Myocardial Ischemia: Effects of Carnitine

James R. Neely, David Garber, Kathleen McDonough, and
Jane Idell-Wenger

*Department of Physiology, Milton S. Hershey Medical Center, Pennsylvania State
University, Hershey, Pennsylvania 17033*

The metabolic and functional consequences of myocardial ischemia have been studied extensively in recent years. From these studies, it has become increasingly clear that cardiac muscle can tolerate rather long periods of total oxygen deprivation and still regain normal mechanical function on reinstitution of oxygen supply. Heart muscle possesses intrinsic mechanisms whereby energy use via muscle contraction is decreased on exposure to low oxygen supply. In addition, such techniques as potassium arrest can preserve energy levels and allow the muscle to withstand total ischemia for periods of 1 hr or more. Nonetheless, after prolonged periods of ischemia, irreversible damage to the cell does occur.

The fact that oxygen lack per se does not result in immediate irreversible damage has led to the concept that alterations in the cellular content of key constituents such as enzymes, metabolites, and metabolic products that occur secondarily to a decrease in oxidative metabolism results in irreversible ischemic damage. Thus, rather than cause irreversible damage, reduced oxidative metabolism probably establishes the condition for otherwise normal cellular processes to eventually destroy the cell. A major consequence of prolonged ischemia that has been observed in a number of laboratories is the loss of total adenine nucleotides from the cell (1). This loss of nucleotides has been related to the onset of irreversible cellular damage (2–5). However, during the course of adenine nucleotide loss, many other events occur which could contribute to death of the myocyte. For example, long-chain acyl CoA and long-chain acyl carnitine levels increase in myocardial ischemia (6), and the accumulation of these compounds in response to decreased oxidative metabolism has been proposed as a mechanism that can result in damage to several enzyme systems in the myocardium (7,8). Accumulation of long-chain acyl CoA and acyl carnitine esters and the relationship of high levels of these compounds to cellular damage to the myocardium have been studied in the isolated perfused rat heart. The results of these studies are discussed.

225

METHODS

Hearts from 200- to 300-g Sprague-Dawley male rats were removed and perfused in the isolated working rat heart preparation as described previously (9). Ischemia was induced by use of a one-way aortic valve that prevents retrograde perfusion of the coronary arteries during diastole. Hypoxia and anoxia were induced by gassing the perfusate with 20 or 0% oxygen. The gas phase contained 5% CO_2 in each case, and the remainder was N_2. Zero flow ischemia was produced by cross-clamping the aortic cannula and decreasing left atrial pressure to zero. The perfusate was Krebs Henseleit bicarbonate buffer containing either glucose or glucose plus fatty acids as substrate. Tissue levels of long-chain acyl CoA and acyl carnitine were determined as previously described (10).

RESULTS AND DISCUSSION

Of the numerous products of metabolism that accumulate in ischemic tissue, probably the first to accumulate is NADH in the mitochondria as a consequence of reduced oxygen as electron acceptor for the electron transport chain. High levels of NADH inhibit several steps in metabolic pathways, one of which is β-oxidation of fatty acids, as shown in Fig. 1. This inhibition of β-oxidation results in the accumulation of long-chain acyl CoA and long-chain acyl carnitine in the mitochondria, and by reduced removal of acyl carnitine from the mitochondrial matrix, levels of long-chain acyl carnitine and probably acyl CoA accumu-

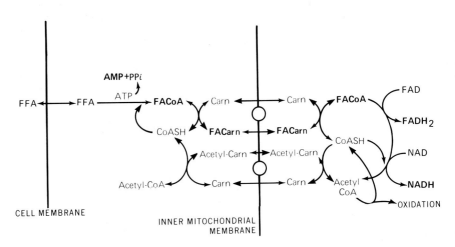

FIG. 1. Schematic representation of NADH inhibition of β-oxidation of long-chain fatty acids. With myocardial ischemia, hypoxia, or anoxia, NADH and $FADH_2$ levels increase in the mitochondria. This results in reduced flux of long-chain acyl CoA (FACoA) through β-oxidation, and its level increases in the mitochondria. The increase in FACoA/CoA ratio causes long-chain acyl carnitine (FACarn) to increase in probably both the mitochondria and cytosol. FACoA and FFA would then be expected to increase in the cytosol.

late in the cytosol (11). This increase in acyl CoA and acyl carnitine has been demonstrated in isolated rat hearts under ischemic and hypoxic conditions (6) and has been reported to occur in models of regional ischemia in the dog (12) and pig heart (13). The extent of accumulation of acyl esters of CoA and carnitine is dependent on the availability of exogenous fatty acid as well as the time of perfusion under ischemic conditions (16).

Both long-chain acyl CoA and acyl carnitine have been proposed as metabolites the abnormal accumulation of which may interfere with normal cellular function. Both compounds inhibit mitochondrial respiration. Acyl CoA inhibits adenine nucleotide translocase in isolated mitochondria, with a reported inhibition coefficient, K_i, value of 0.15 μM (14). However, this K_i value for extramitochondrial acyl CoA is dependent on the acyl CoA/mitochondrial protein ratio (15). At ratios of acyl CoA/mitochondrial protein that would exist in the intact cell, cytosolic acyl CoA would never accumulate to levels expected to inhibit adenine nucleotide translocase. Approximately 95% of the total CoA is located in the mitochondria matrix, and accumulation of acyl CoA during ischemia is predominantly in the mitochondria (11). Using mitochondrial particles with the matrix surface of the inner membranes exposed to the incubation medium, acyl CoA has been shown to inhibit adenine nucleotide translocase by competing with adenine nucleotides on the inner surface of the inner mitochondrial membrane (14). However, as reported recently, accumulation of acyl CoA in the matrix of intact isolated mitochondria does not inhibit adenine nucleotide translocase to any significant extent (15).

Fatty acyl carnitine has been reported to inhibit a number of enzyme systems. High concentrations of acyl carnitine added to isolated mitochondria inhibit oxidative metabolism of these mitochondria, as demonstrated in Table 1. The

TABLE 1. *Effects of palmityl carnitine on mitochondrial respiration*[a]

Palmityl carnitine (nmoles/mg)	pH	O_2 consumption (natoms/min/mg)	
		State 4	State 3
0	7.4	69	406
18		50	392
27		57	359
48		57	302
63		58	282
86		57	248
114		73	158
0	6.5	58	319
25		49	237
48		54	221

[a] Mitochondria were isolated from rat hearts as described previously (11). State 3 respiration rates were determined by addition of ADP following 1 min incubation with palmityl carnitine at the levels indicated.

data in this table indicate that acyl carnitine does not interfere with state 4 respiratory rates, but reduces state 3 rates. A significant inhibition was observed at 27 nmoles palmityl carnitine per milligram mitochondrial protein. The maximal ratio of palmityl carnitine/mitochondrial protein that can accumulate in ischemic tissue is 16 nmoles/mg. This suggests that acyl carnitine most likely would not interfere with respiration of ischemic tissue. A decrease in the medium pH had an inhibitory effect on state 3 rates (see Table 1), and acyl carnitine was more effective as an inhibitor of oxidation at the lower pH. Thus, a combination of low cellular pH and high acyl carnitine in ischemic cells could interfere with residual respiration. Acyl carnitine has also been demonstrated to inhibit calcium uptake of sarcoplasmic reticulum (16,17) and sarcoplasmic sodium potassium ATPase (18). Free fatty acids also inhibit sodium potassium ATPase (19). In addition to the inhibition of specific enzyme systems, these compounds are good detergents and may affect the function of many enzymes and membranes in a nonspecific way.

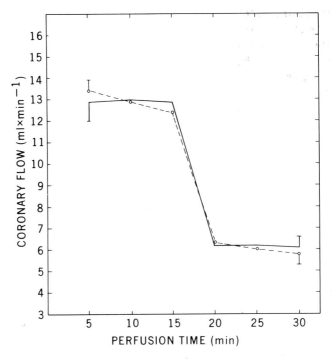

FIG. 2. Coronary flow in control and ischemic rat hearts. Hearts were perfused for 10 min as a Langendorf preparation with a 60 mm Hg perfusion pressure and with buffer containing glucose (11 mM). At zero time in the figure, they were switched to working hearts with a left atrial pressure of 10 cm H_2O. The perfusate was Krebs bicarbonate buffer containing either 11 mM glucose and 1.5 mM U-^{14}C-palmitate bound to 3% BSA *(solid line)* or the same substrate with 4 mM DL-carnitine *(dashed line)*. Control perfusion was continued for 15 min, at which time coronary flow was reduced by approximately 60% for an additional 15 min ischemic perfusion.

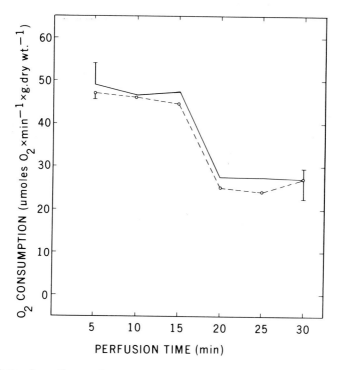

FIG. 3. Effects of carnitine on O_2 consumption during control and ischemic perfusion. Data were obtained from the same hearts as in Fig. 2. *Solid line* is without and *dashed line* is with 4 mM D,L-carnitine.

Because the potential exists for acyl CoA to interfere with oxidative metabolism in ischemic myocardium, it has been proposed that addition of exogenous carnitine to ischemic tissue should improve myocardial metabolism and function by lowering acyl CoA (20). Infusion of carnitine into the ischemic zone of a dog heart model of regional ischemia was reported to improve the electrical changes that occur during ischemia (20). Addition of carnitine in ischemic pig heart improved regional mechanical motion (21). If carnitine is to be effective in relieving the accumulation of acyl CoA, exogenous carnitine must get into the ischemic cells and it must be demonstrated that the level of acyl CoA decreases. The cellular level of carnitine decreased in both the dog and pig models of ischemia, suggesting that carnitine is lost from ischemic tissue and that exogenous carnitine might be beneficial. In addition, exogenous carnitine lowered the level of acyl CoA and increased the level of acyl carnitine in ischemic pig hearts receiving high levels of fatty acid (21). These studies with carnitine were repeated in the ischemic rat heart preparation and no beneficial effects of carnitine could be demonstrated.

Figure 2 illustrates that coronary flow was unaltered by carnitine and Fig. 3 illustrates that the rate of oxygen consumption was the same in ischemic

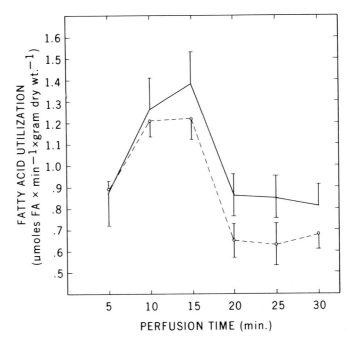

FIG. 4. Fatty acid oxidation. Data obtained from same hearts as in Fig. 2. Perfusion with U-^{14}C-palmitate (1.5 mM) was started at zero time. By 15 min of control perfusion, the rate of $^{14}CO_2$ production had increased to a steady state indicating that the specific activity of citric acid cycle intermediates had approached that of the perfusate fatty acid. Induction of ischemia at 15 min greatly reduced fatty acid oxidation.

hearts with and without carnitine present. Figure 4 demonstrates that the rate of fatty acid oxidation was not influenced by the presence of exogenous carnitine, and Fig. 5 illustrates that carnitine was ineffective in improving ventricular function either in the control or ischemic heart. In fact, those hearts receiving 4 mM DL-carnitine showed a slight reduction in ventricular performance. In addition, the presence of extracellular carnitine did not alter the accumulation of acyl carnitine or acyl CoA in the tissue (Table 2), and normal rat hearts perfused with buffer containing 10 mM carnitine did not show a net increase in the intracellular concentration of carnitine (Table 3).

These data demonstrate that net carnitine uptake by the rat heart is either extremely slow or nonexistent and that addition of exogenous carnitine does not alter the intracellular concentration of carnitine in either control or ischemic hearts; neither was the accumulation of long-chain acyl CoA and acyl carnitine altered in ischemic hearts. The data from the rat heart as compared to dog and pig hearts indicate that there is either a species difference in the response of ischemic myocardium to carnitine or that carnitine is ineffective in altering the metabolism of ischemic cardiac muscle. It is possible that the reported beneficial effects of carnitine on electrical activity and on regional mechanical

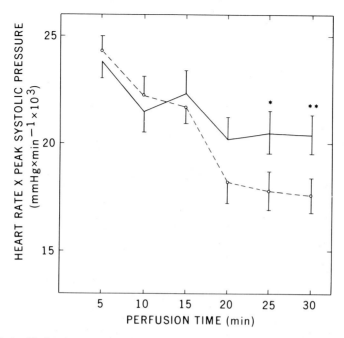

FIG. 5. Effects of ischemia and carnitine on ventricular function. Data for peak systolic pressure and heart rate were obtained from the hearts described in Fig. 2. Ventricular function decreased slightly more during ischemic perfusion with carnitine present in the perfusate. *, $p < 0.05$; **, $p < 0.025$.

motion in the dog and pig are related to properties of carnitine other than its ability to alter acyl CoA levels in the tissue.

Another observation that indicates that long-chain acyl CoA and acyl carnitine may have only minimal effects on ischemic tissue is provided by a comparison of the tissue levels of these acyl esters in hearts under a variety of oxygen-deficient conditions, as shown in Table 4. Both acyl CoA and acyl carnitine increased to quite high levels in ischemic, hypoxic, and anoxic hearts even

TABLE 2. *Effects of exogenous carnitine on tissue levels of acyl CoA and acyl carnitine in ischemic hearts[a]*

Condition	Acyl carnitine	Acyl CoA
Control	498 ± 159	99 ± 8
Ischemic	$3,874 \pm 175$	270 ± 17
Ischemic + carnitine	$4,164 \pm 376$	265 ± 13

[a]The perfusate contained glucose (11 mM) and palmitate (1.5 mM bound to 3% BSA). Perfusion was continued for 15 min either as control (normal coronary flow), ischemic (coronary flow 50% of control), or ischemic with DL-carnitine (4 mM) added to the perfusate.

TABLE 3. *Effects of exogenous carnitine on intracellular carnitine in control hearts*[a]

Perfusate L-carnitine (mM)	Total intracellular carnitine (nmoles/g dry wt)
0	6,750 ± 240
10	6,200 ± 105

[a] Control hearts were perfused for 20 min with perfusate containing either 0 or 10 mM L-carnitine. Total intracellular levels were determined by measuring total tissue free carnitine after hydrolysis at pH 12 for 1 hr to break down all acyl carnitines. Extracellular carnitine was substrated from the total by measuring sorbitol space and perfusate carnitine.

though the rates of coronary flow and work output of these hearts was quite different. However, when perfused hearts were maintained for 10 min with zero flow, as indicated by autolysis in Table 4, the level of acyl CoA increased, but the level of acyl carnitine remained unchanged.

The time-course of changes in acyl CoA and acyl carnitine in rat hearts incubated at 37°C demonstrates that the level of both acyl esters decreases with time in autolysing myocardium (Table 5). This rather surprising observation indicates that the levels of acyl CoA and acyl carnitine do not increase under all conditions of ischemia in which cellular damage is known to occur. Thus, it would appear that cellular deterioration and irreversible damage which is known to occur in autolysing tissue can occur in the absence of high levels of acyl CoA and acyl carnitine, again suggesting that the effects of these compounds in ischemic myocardium is minimal. We have recently reported that a faster

TABLE 4. *Long-chain acyl CoA and carnitine derivatives in hearts under various conditions of oxygen deficiency*[a]

Condition	C.F. (ml/min)	P.S.P. × hr (mm Hg/min × 10³)	FACoA (nmoles/g dry wt)	FACarn (nmoles/g dry wt)
Control	28 ± 0.6	36	99 ± 8	498 ± 159
Ischemic	2 ± 0.3	6	240 ± 29	2,428 ± 137
Hypoxic	22 ± 0.9	15	288 ± 10	3,533 ± 188
Anoxic	19 ± 2	10	286 ± 7	3,192 ± 259
Autolysis	—	—	210 ± 13	600 ± 99

[a] Hearts were perfused for 10 min as Langendorff preparations with buffer containing glucose (11 mM) and gassed with 95% O_2 and 5% CO_2. They were then switched to the working preparation and perfused with buffer containing glucose (11 mM) and palmitate (1.0 mM bound to 3% BSA) for an additional 5 min. The perfusion was then continued for 10 min with the same buffer gassed with 95% O_2, 5% CO_2 (controls and ischemic); 20% O_2, 5% CO_2 and 75% N_2 (hypoxic); or 95% N_2, 5% CO_2 (anoxic); or perfusion was stopped by clamping the aortic outflow tube and left atrial input tube for 10 min (autolysis). The hearts were quick frozen with Wollenberg clamps and assayed for long-chain acyl CoA (FACoA) and acyl carnitine (FACarn).

TABLE 5. *Effect of incubation time on tissue long-chain acyl CoA and acyl carnitine in autolyzing tissue*[a]

Incubation time (min)	FACoA (nmoles/g dry wt)	FACarn (nmoles/g dry wt)
0	175 ± 19	141 ± 87
5	146 ± 13	65 ± 27
10	111 ± 4	15 ± 8
15	102 ± 19	7 ± 4
30	87 ± 4	0.32 ± 0.3
60	122 ± 12	32 ± 15

[a]Hearts were removed from rats and the ventricles trimmed free of atria, washed with saline, and incubated at 37°C in 50-ml flasks for the times indicated.

rate of ventricular failure in hearts from diabetic animals exposed to severe ischemic conditions was associated with higher tissue levels of acyl CoA and acyl carnitine (22).

SUMMARY

In summary, the response of ischemic myocardium to addition of exogenous carnitine may show a species specificity. Dog and pig heart appear to respond with improved electrical and mechanical function, whereas exogenous carnitine has no effect on the rat heart. Both the dog and pig heart lose cellular carnitine during the course of ischemia, whereas the rat heart does not. Addition of exogenous carnitine to the ischemic pig heart lowers tissue levels of acyl CoA and increases tissue levels of acyl carnitine. In the rat heart, exogenous carnitine does not affect the levels of either of these acyl esters, nor does it increase the intracellular level of free carnitine. Thus it would appear that exogenous carnitine is without effect in the ischemic rat heart.

REFERENCES

1. Neely, J. R., Rovetto, M. J., Whitmer, J. T., and Morgan, H. E. (1973): Effects of ischemia on ventricular function and metabolism in the isolated working rat heart, *Am. J. Physiol.*, 225:651–658.
2. Gudbjarnason, S., Mathes, P., and Ravens, K. G. (1920): Functional compartmentation of ATP and creatine phosphate in heart muscle. *J. Mol. Cell. Cardiol.*, 1:325–339.
3. Kübler, W., and Spieckermann, P. G. (1970): Regulation of glycolysis in the ischemic and anoxic myocardium. *J. Mol. Cell. Cardiol.*, 1:351–377.
4. Wollenberger, A., and Krause, E. G. (1968): Metabolic characteristics of the acutely ischemic myocardium. *Am. J. Cardiol.*, 22:349–359.
5. Reibel, D. K., and Rovetto, M. J. (1978): Myocardial ATP synthesis and mechanical function following oxygen deficiency. *Am. J. Physiol.*, 234(5):H620–H624.
6. Whitmer, J. T., Wenger, J. I., Rovetto, M. J., and Neely, J. R. (1978): Control of fatty acid metabolism in hypoxic and ischemic hearts. *J. Biol. Chem.*, 253:4305–4309.
7. Opie, L. H. (1979): Role of carnitine in fatty acid metabolism of normal and ischemic myocardium. *Am. Heart J.*, 97:375–388.

8. Shug, A. L., Shrago, E., and Bittar, N. (1975): Acyl-CoA inhibition of adenine nucleotide translocation in ischemic myocardium. *Am. J. Physiol.,* 228:689–692.
9. Neely, J. R., Liebermeister, H., Battersby, E. J., and Morgan, H. E. (1967): Effect of pressure development on oxygen consumption by isolated rat heart. *Am. J. Physiol.,* 212:804–814.
10. Oram, J. F., Bennetch, S. L., and Neely, J. R. (1973): Regulation of fatty acid utilization in isolated perfused rat hearts. *J. Biol. Chem.,* 248:5299–5309.
11. Idell-Wenger, J. A., Grotyohann, L. W., and Neely, J. R. (1978): Coenzyme A and carnitine distribution in normal and ischemic hearts. *J. Biol. Chem.,* 253:4310–4318.
12. Shug, A. L., Thomsen, J. H., Folts, J. D., Bittar, N., Klein, M. E., Koke, J. R., and Huth, P. J. (1978): Changes in tissue levels of carnitine and other metabolites during myocardial ischemia and anoxia. *Arch. Biochem. Biophys.,* 187:25–33.
13. Liedtke, A. J., Nellis, S., and Neely, J. R. (1978): Effects of excess free fatty acids on mechanical and metabolic function in normal and ischemic myocardium. *Circ. Res.,* 43:652–661.
14. Chua, B., and Shrago, E. (1977): Reversible inhibition of adenine nucleotide translocation by long chain acyl-CoA esters in bovine heart mitochondria and inverted submitochondrial particles. Comparison with atractylate and bongkrekic acid. *J. Biol. Chem.,* 252:6711–6714.
15. Watts, J. A., Koch, C. D., and LaNoue, K. F. (1979): Adenine nucleotide transport during cardiac ischemia. *Am. J. Physiol. (submitted).*
16. Pitts, B. J. R., Tate, C. A., Von Winkle, W. B., Entman, M. L., and Wood, J. M. (1978): Palmityl carnitine inhibition of the calcium pump in cardiac sarcoplasmic reticulum: A possible role in myocardial ischemia. *Life Sci.,* 23:391–402.
17. Cohen, D., Wang, T., Sumida, M., Adams, R., Tsi, L. I., Grupp, G., and Schwartz, A. (1978): Effect of palmitylcarnitine on cardiac and skeletal sarcoplasmic reticulum (abstr.). *Fed. Proc.,* 37:376.
18. Wood, J. M., Bush, B., Pitts, B. J. R., and Schwartz, A. (1977): Inhibition of bovine heart Na^+, K^+-ATPase by palmitylcarnitine and palmityl-CoA. *Biochem. Biophys. Res. Commun.,* 74:677–684.
19. Lamers, J. M. J., and Hülsmann, W. C. (1977): Inhibition of ($Na^+ + K^+$)-stimulated ATPase of heart by fatty acids. *J. Mol. Cell. Cardiol.,* 9:343–346.
20. Folts, J. D., Shug, A. L., Koke, J. R., and Bittar, P. (1978): Protection of the ischemic dog myocardium with carnitine. *Am. J. Cardiol.,* 41:1209–1214.
21. Liedtke, A. J., and Nellis, S. H. (1979): Effects of carnitine in ischemic and fatty acid supplemented swine hearts. *J. Clin. Invest. (in press).*
22. Feuvray, D., Idell-Wenger, J. A., and Neely, J. R. (1979): Effects of ischemia on rat myocardial function and metabolism in diabetes. *Circ. Res.,* 44:322–329.

Ischemic Myocardium and Antianginal Drugs,
edited by M. M. Winbury and Y. Abiko.
Raven Press, New York © 1979.

Discussion: Metabolic Changes

Richard J. Bing, *Chairman*

Bing: Dr. Imai, you have described what occurs in global ischemia. Is the ischemia reversible? If you have a long period of ischemia and reperfusion, will everything turn out all right? Most of the data that I have seen show that ATP is replenished. My specific question is this: Does not the effect of reperfusion depend on the initial damage that has been done? Is it related to the severity and duration of ischemia?

Imai: As far as the mechanical performance is concerned, it is reversible even after 40 min of ischemia, but the ATP level does not return to the control level even after 15 min of reperfusion. We found a significant difference between the ATP content after 40 min of ischemia and that after 1 or 5 min of ischemia. So there was a difference in the ATP level after reperfusion depending on the duration of ischemia.

J. Schaper: We did almost the same study in the isolated dog heart with global ischemia and measured various parameters, including ATP and phosphocreatine levels; and we did ultrastructure investigations of the same tissue and measured the function of the heart during the reperfusion period. I agree with Dr. Imai that the decline in the ATP content is indicative of the severity of ischemic injury but not of the ability of the tissue to recover. For that, you need to measure the phosphocreatine content. As long as phosphocreatine is going up, everything is all right and the injury is reversible.

Bing: Shall we go to Dr. Opie's report about the role of cyclic AMP?

Hashimoto: Dr. Opie, does the cyclic AMP level increase during ischemia? How many minutes of ischemia are necessary to increase the tissue cyclic AMP level?

Opie: This depends on the model used. The data I showed were only in the baboon model. If you use other models, you can get other patterns of cyclic AMP rise.

Hashimoto: I am just thinking of the electrophysiology. The sodium channel is immediately inactivated and then the calcium current begins. This means that the vulnerable period is connected with the relationship between the sodium and calcium ions. Therefore, I wonder if ischemia increases the amount of free calcium in the cell. The calcium may act on the adenyl cyclase to increase the cyclic AMP level, and it may also activate the sodium current. By my understanding, there is no direct connection between the cyclic AMP level and the decrease of the fibrillation threshold, but free calcium in the ischemic tissue may increase adenyl cyclase and open the sodium channel.

Opie: Thank you very much for that comment because it might have appeared that we believe there is a simple relationship between cyclic AMP and the ion movements, and obviously there is not. We think calcium ion movements may be important in the setting of the ischemia. We believe that the very rapid rise in extracellular potassium, which Dr. Henry has commented about to me personally, inhibits the sodium channel; and, under those conditions, cyclic AMP can promote the slow response, which is calcium dependent. But there must be an inhibition of the fast channel, which we believe is mediated by potassium in ischemia. I would also like to say that even this is an oversimplification because cyclic AMP presumably acts on the calcium channel by protein kinase phosphorylation. However, protein kinase has not yet been identified and its phosphorylation has not yet been proved, so this is speculation. If I may just add briefly that, clearly, as Dr. Wollenberger pointed out earlier this week, we are dealing in most of these phosphorylation events with the balance between cyclic AMP and cyclic GMP. It is a serious deficiency of our hypothesis that we are unable thus far to report data on cyclic GMP or on the presumably antagonistic effect of cyclic AMP and GMP.

Bing: Any further discussion on this subject? You really are very careful, Lionel, in speculating on the reasons for the relationship between fibrillation and cyclic AMP. What do you think is the most likely link?

Opie: Well, in ischemia, I believe we can construct a reasonable chain of events. As I have just outlined, the high level of potassium is inhibiting the fast channel. But, in our perfused heart preparation, the whole perfused heart is not ischemic and has normal ATP and normal phosphocreatine, so I cannot invoke that explanation. I can only say that Dr. Tada from Osaka passed on to me the information that they had an article suggesting that increased intracellular calcium current in normal heart, can, in some circumstances, mediate an increased intracellular potassium and have a similar effect on the action potential. If this is so, it might explain our findings, but I really do not know if it works in a normal heart.

Bing: Does phosphodiesterase inhibition favor the onset of fibrillation?

Opie: That is right. That is exactly what you expect. I am trying to persuade somebody from a pharmaceutical company to make me a phosphodiesterase activator that might have therapeutic and antiarrhythmic qualities. But so far, nobody has been interested in that.

Hashimoto: Does a change in pH affect the phosphodiesterase activity?

Opie: Yes. Phosphodiesterase is very sensistive to pH and, as the pH falls from about 7 down to 6.5, one would expect phosphodiesterase inhibition to occur and cyclic AMP to build up.

Bing: Dr. Gudbjarnason, there is one question that occurred to me when I looked at your data. How can you be so sure where the free fatty acids come from? Do they come from phospholipids or from glycerides? For example, in myocardial infarction, I always thought that free fatty acids came from inhibition of acyl CoA transferase in the mitochondrial membrane.

Gudbjarnason: The free fatty acid composition of triglycerides is very different from that of phospholipids. Phospholipids contain polyunsaturated fatty acids, whereas one of the determinants of glycerides is oleic acid and more saturated fatty acids. We compared the composition of glycerides, phospholipids, and free fatty acid fractions. Under normal conditions and in most cases of accidental deaths, we estimated that 80% of the free fatty acids found came from phospholipid breakdown and about 20% from triglycerides. From the sample composition, you can make an educated guess as to the primary source of these free fatty acids. In those cases, with extremely high levels of free fatty acids, the free fatty acids have the composition of glycerides. They are probably from the blood and do not resemble the free fatty acids released by autolysis from the muscle itself.

Bing: Yes, I understand. I was just thinking of labeling phospholipids and then recovering the label in the free fatty acids, thereby demonstrating beyond a shadow of a doubt where the free fatty acids come from. Is that possible?

Gudbjarnason: This could be done in experimental animals. Dr. Wecklike did similar studies a few years ago. Isolated rat hearts were perfused and the release of individual fatty acids determined. In ischemic hearts, there was a very early breakdown of certain phospholipids. He also made an interesting observation on the different stability of individual phospholipids. Phosphatidyl ethanolamines were more unstable than the phosphatidyl cholines. That agrees with our observations.

Nakamura: Dr. Gudbjarnason, if you produced an ischemia, how fast could you expect the change of fatty acid composition of phospholipids in the myocardium to occur?

Gudbjarnason: The only way we attempted to produce relative ischemia was to use the isoproterenol model. Then we killed the animals ½, 1, 2, and 48 hr after the injection of these very large doses of isoproterenol. We already saw significant changes after 30 min.

Nakamura: Does this mean that significant changes were produced before the occurrence of necrosis?

Gudbjarnason: Yes, and we could also see similar adaptive changes when we used norepinephrine. In these cases, we did not observe necrotic lesions. There are several changes that took place that seem to be adaptive and not associated with necrotic lesions.

Nakamura: Do you also expect it when the coronary artery is occluded?

Gudbjarnason: We did observe similar changes in human heart muscle with severe coronary artery stenosis, but it was unexpected to see the low level of free fatty acids in human hearts with severe coronary artery stenosis. The FFA was much lower than expected and was lower than what we observed in accidental death cases and in certain deaths without coronary atherosclerosis. This brings up the question of carnitine and the efforts to influence lipolysis. If you are attempting to modify the free fatty acids in the infarct, the heart itself has made arrangements to lower lipolysis during some phase of adaptation. We do not find any evidence of very high levels of FFA in human coronary artery occlusion and myocardial infarction. And I think the whole question of correlation between the plasma level and the tissue level has not been clarified. Dr. Bing showed 25 years ago that there was a correlation between the myocardial uptake of free fatty acids and the arterial concentration; there is a saturation point. What determines the saturation point is not really known, whether it is esterification or oxidation. But it has not been estimated what level of FFA there is normally in an intact myocardium and how much FFA can be tolerated.

Nakamura: This means that an experimental coronary occlusion study has not been done, is that correct?

Gudbjarnason: Dr. Bing was showing earlier today an experimental occlusion; there is an increase in free fatty acid level. But is that really reflecting what we see in atherosclerosis in the human heart?

Bing: No; the experimental occlusion is an acute infarction, and a chronic situation may be very different.

Gudbjarnason: I suspect that what we are seeing in an atherosclerotic human heart is an adaptive change and a diminution of lipolytic activity. We find low myocardial levels of FFA consistently in those with atherosclerosis, and most of these have myocardial infarction.

Nakamura: I am asking about fresh and acute infarction.

Gudbjarnason: Many of the infarcts are acute, but these hearts have severe coronary artery stenosis.

Henry: I would like to ask if you would speculate on the potential importance of lysophospholipids that could be generated during ischemia. The detergent effect of these compounds has recently been shown to be very membrane active and to alter the monophasic action potential of Purkinje fibers.

Gudbjarnason: I think these lysolipids are quite important. We look for them, and the amount we find is relatively low, probably because degradation has gone far beyond the lysolipid stage by the time we get the autopsy material. There may be a much larger quantity initially, but there are no large quantities by the time we get autopsy samples. It is well known from various membrane systems that lysolipids are very membranolytic. The abnormal glycerides that we find accumulating in a human ischemic heart or at least in hearts with severe coronary stenosis have a composition that resembles the composition of phospholipids and not that of normal triglycerides. This could be due to phospholipase C activity and removal of the polar heads. It is known from ischemia in the brain that this can occur. Then diglycerides sit in the membrane, and there they can change the membrane morphology and possibly the membrane function. I think this could explain the abnormal glyceride composition we find in the human heart.

Bing: May I ask Dr. Opie one more question? Dr. Schwarz has now stated that the calcium antagonists inhibit adenyl cyclase. Are you familiar with that work?

Opie: Calcium antagonists inhibit adenyl cyclase?

Bing: Yes, he said that one thing calcium antagonists have in common is that they inhibit adenyl cyclase.

Opie: How did he show that?

Bing: It was just an observation.

Opie: Well, at the moment, I am impressed by the size of the beta-blockade effect by the nonspecific nature of antiarrhythmic agents in decreasing cyclic AMP, and they presumably do this by inhibiting adenyl cyclase. So I think that this is a phenomenon that has not been well explored at all.

Overview

Ischemic Myocardium and Antianginal Drugs,
edited by M. M. Winbury and Y. Abiko.
Raven Press, New York © 1979.

Overview

Lionel H. Opie

MRC Ischaemic Heart Disease Research Unit, Department of Medicine, Groote Schuur Hospital and University of Cape Town Medical School, 7925 Cape Town, South Africa

It is now my task to summarize the highlights of this volume. You will see that most of the important problems concerning the metabolism and pharmacology of the ischemic myocardium have been discussed.

A fundamental problem in the consideration of ischemia is the nature and timing of the *"point of no return."* Although in their study *J. Schaper et al.* were looking for the point of no return, they found that perhaps there was no clear point of no return. Forty-five minutes of coronary artery occlusion produced severe changes, and Schaper et al. were able to show that different pathological changes occurred even in adjacent cells, some of which were moderately and some of which were irreversibly damaged. Their data, and those of W. Schaper, seemed to support the concept of very steep gradients of oxygen in the border zone.

But does the *border zone* really exist? Here I would like to digress to refer to some collaborative work with Hearse et al. (6). We took multiple biopsies across the edge of a developing dog infarct about 25 min after ligation and found a gradual fall of the value of ATP across the visible border (Fig. 1), with a narrow border zone of 6 mm (6); there was a similar pattern for lactate (Fig. 2), with a border zone of 8 mm. Thus, there would be the same pattern for NADH accumulation and, therefore, there would be exactly the same pattern for the nitrobluetetrazolium stain (NBT) because loss of NBT staining is no longer apparent when NAD is added to incubated heart tissue (10). Thus, the NBT staining would be lost as NADH accumulated, and depending on the sensitivity of the NBT reaction, there might be a vary sharp border even if tissue NADH increased less rapidly. Therefore, there might be a difference between a sharp NBT border, as found by W. Schaper, and the biochemically measured metabolic border zone.

However, this is not to say that there must of necessity be a border zone. Chance (3) made some very provocative comments at a meeting in Dallas in 1976. He believed that mitochondria responded to oxygen in an on–off way. Thus, mitochondria were either not working at all or working flat-out and, therefore, the border for oxygen would be extremely sharp and might even be

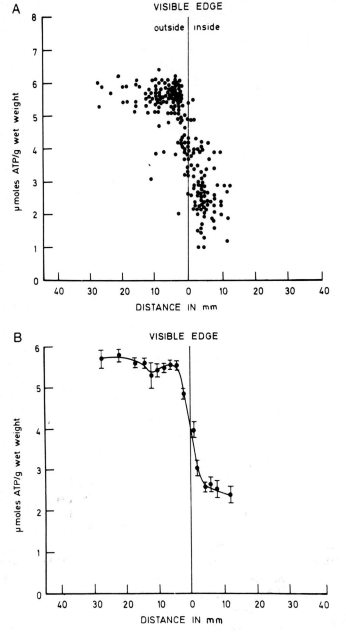

FIG. 1. Linear changes of tissue adenosine triphosphate *(ATP)* concentration in relation to the edge of the visible area of cyanosis *(central vertical line on each graph),* with tissue samples obtained from outside the area of cyanosis plotted to the *left* of center and tissue samples obtained from inside the area of cyanosis plotted to the *right* of center, observed between 21 and 26 min after coronary artery ligation. **A:** Individual data points obtained from all experiments plotted as µmoles ATP/g wet weight recorded in samples against the distance of each sample in millimeters from the edge of the visible area of necrosis. **B:** The statistical mean of the results ($n = 230$ biopsy sites). *Bar* indicates SEM. (From Hearse et al., ref 6; reproduced by permission of the *American Journal of Cardiology.*)

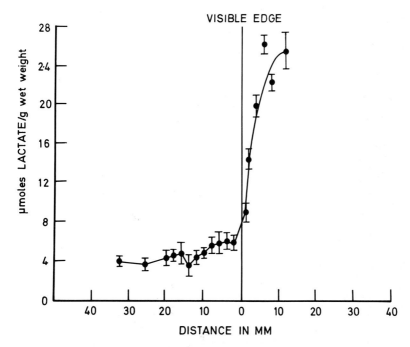

FIG. 2. Linear changes of tissue lactate concentration in relation to the edge of the visible area of cyanosis. For representional details, see legend to Fig. 1. (From Hearse et al., ref. 6; reproduced by permission of the *American Journal of Cardiology.*)

a border between adjacent mitochondria. Chance's concepts have been supported by subsequent experimental work (14). But these data do not imply that there is no wider border for metabolism. A model can be constructed (Fig. 3) in which two mitochondria would be working in an on–off way (one on, one off), rather than at half-speed during oxygen deprivation (3,11), but the net effect would still be half the required ATP production in either case. Thus there could still be graded effects on glycolysis and a mixed metabolic pattern, with an apparent border zone. So it may well be, as Chance suggested, that there is a different border for glycolysis than there is for oxygen. At the moment, several very interesting publications are coming from the laboratories of Chance, Williamson, and their co-workers. But they are using NADH fluorescence as a marker of the border zone, and NADH fluorescence may not be sensitive enough to detect intermediate changes; NADH fluorescence may be an on–off indicator. Furthermore, as *W. Schaper* pointed out, it is the smaller infarcts that have the more obvious "twilight zone" of jeopardized myocardium. It is not yet known if infarcts found in patients have an early "border zone."

Consideration of the border zone also brings us to the difficulty of the *biochemical assessment of irreversibility. J. Schaper et al.* clearly showed that low ATP (as low as 1 μmole/g wet wt) by itself does not indicate irreversibility

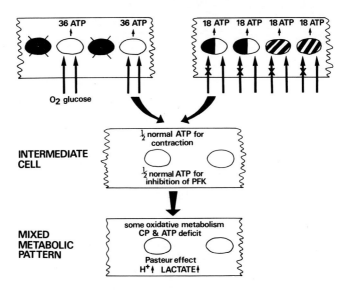

FIG. 3. Two schematic heart cells are shown. In both, the supply of O_2 and substrate (glucose in this case) are reduced by half. *Left,* a cell in which alternate mitochondria *(white)* are working with other anoxic mitochondria not working *(black with crosses). Right,* each mitochondrion is only working at half-capacity *(half black, half white).* In either model, effectively only half the mitochondria are functioning, only half the normal ATP is made, a deficit of ATP and creatine phosphate (CP) arises, phosphofructokinase (PFK) inhibition is decreased, and a Pasteur effect may be expected. If both ischemic and hypoxic, the cell will also accumulate H^+ and lactate. This model argues for the existence of an "intermediate cell," one that is neither anoxic nor normoxic. (From Opie, ref. 11; reproduced by permission of the American Heart Association.)

[in contrast to the concept that there can be a critical point of no return (8,9) with ATP levels that are much higher]. That changes in total ATP should not always correlate with irreversibility is in accord with the speculative concept of compartmentation of cellular ATP and, in particular, the possible role of glycolytically produced ATP in the preservation of the cell membrane (2).

Another proposed biochemical cause of irreversibility is the development of *tissue acidosis,* which was studied by *Ichihara et al.* They used a pH-sensitive electrode to assess the development of tissue acidosis after coronary ligation in the dog. The pH drop after ligation was inhibited by β blockade. A very interesting fundamental observation was that the pH fall was sensitive to β blockade, whereas the lactate rise was not. There are theoretical reasons for supposing that proton production during glycolysis is not the product of lactate production, but is instead the product of simultaneous ATP breakdown and turnover (5). The direct products of anaerobic glycolysis are lactate and ATP; and the eventual products are lactate, ADP, and protons. The data of Ichihara et al. are probably the first to show a difference between the behavior of lactate and of protons. But to validate their results fully, Ichihara et al. would be advised to use an enzymatic determination of lactate.

Another factor in irreversibility of ischemic damage may be changes in water permeability [see Whalen et al. (15)]. *Koyama et al.* presented novel data on *colloid osmotic pressure* changes in ischemia; the rapidity of changes in colloid osmotic pressure found in their study was indeed surprising. If such changes were associated with irreversible injury [as suggested by data on changes in water permeability of ischemic cells (15)], then Koyama et al. were beginning to detect something irreversible happening very early and within 2 min. I did wonder if perhaps Koyama et al. were liberating enzymes in their reperfusion system and if this was contributing to the measurement of the colloid osmotic pressure. Perhaps colloid osmotic pressure changes are not only an index of water flux but also of other factors such as enzyme release.

Another fundamental feature in the production of irreversible ischemic injury is the severity and duration of *oxygen deprivation*. It is reasonable to suppose that antianginal drugs may act by increasing the tissue oxygen tension in the ischemic zone. Winbury has pioneered the use of tissue *oxygen tension measurements* in the assessment of *nitrate* action. Although tissue oxygen tension data are generally held to be controversial, Winbury's data have been fundamental. The chapter by *Winbury and Howe* described the differences between the endocardial and epicardial oxygen tension. During ischemia, endocardial Po_2 falls more than epicardial (16), and nitrates tend to reverse this abnormality. Winbury and Howe described the relationship during ischemia and reperfusion between the fall in oxygen tension and in the changes in hydrogen clearance; the latter is an index of tissue perfusion. The question of the comparative effects of partial and complete release of coronary artery occlusion was also discussed. The critical point is that, when there is a partial release of a coronary ligation, the epicardial but not the endocardial oxygen tension returns to normal but the extent of reactive hyperemia is not normal, which indicates an imperfect degree of reflow. Only total release of the occlusion allowed complete reversal to normal and the full pattern of reactive hyperemia to be completed. The latter phenomenon may be an index of the capacity of the coronary arteries to respond to other vasodilating stimuli, such as exercise. Clinically, the equivalent situation may be that patients with fixed coronary stenosis from coronary artery disease cannot increase their coronary flow adequately in response to exercise, and angina results. A reservation to studies with single-point coronary occlusion is that it is not only the severity of coronary stenosis but also the length of the stenosis that determines the amount of ischemia produced (4).

Yet another factor in the production of irreversible injury is abnormal entry of *calcium ions* into the ischemic cells. Ca^{2+}-antagonist drugs may, therefore, have a fundamental anti-ischemic effect besides acting as coronary vasodilators.

The chapter by *Ono and Hashimoto* examined the controversial question of the comparative effects of various *calcium-antagonist agents*. I am not entirely sure that there are sufficient data to allow us to reach a clear decision on these matters. The issue is complex because calcium antagonists may also have additional effects on Na^+ and K^+ ion movements. Ono and Hashimoto showed that the different calcium-antagonist agents do have very different effects, and they emphasized that, when comparing these agents, it is very important to separate the chronotropic, inotropic, dromotropic, and blood flow effects. Thus, in their model of the excised blood-perfused dog heart, verapamil had only 1/13 of the negative inotropic effect of nifedipine, diltiazem 1/40, and perhexiline 1/100. On the other hand, nifedipine had the smallest effect on atrioventricular conduction and the maximal effect on coronary circulation.

Comparative studies of various Ca^{2+} antagonists to reveal their mode of action at a subcellular level would be very instructive. Furthermore, since the role of *catecholamines* in exaggerating and possibly provoking ischemia is well established, β-blocking agents must be compared with nitrates and calcium antagonists.

Bing et al. provided a new and important general analysis of the mode of action of *antianginal agents.* They considered three groups: those that act on heart volume and coronary flow, β-blocking agents, and calcium antagonists. In the first group, nitrates reduce the volume of the heart, decrease the left ventricular end-diastolic pressure, and, therefore, increase the coronary blood flow; molsidomin has similar but longer-lasting effects. In the second group, although β-antagonist agents may not alter contractility and heart rate, they may alter the relative utilization of glucose and of free fatty acids by the ischemic dog heart (12). In man, β blockade improves lactate uptake by the heart during pacing-induced angina but decreases glucose uptake (7); hence, free fatty acid uptake (not measured in that study) is probably decreased.

These substrate effects are of particular interest because (a) it was the pioneering work of Bing on the substrate metabolism of the human heart that first defined the roles of glucose and fatty acids as myocardial fuels (1); and (b) "oxygen wastage" by fatty acids may play an important role in determining the oxygen uptake during catecholamine stimulation in patients with ischemic heart disease (13).

In the third group of agents, calcium antagonists such as diltiazem have numerous metabolic effects in ischemia: there is a smaller fall of ATP and a smaller rise of lactate, and total tissue free fatty acid is markedly reduced. Different calcium antagonists may have different metabolic effects. Bing et al. found that the ischemic inhibition of glycolysis was relieved by the calcium-antagonist drugs, as shown by the decreased contents of tissue hexosemonophosphates (i.e., glucose-6-phosphate and fructose-6-phosphate). At the same time, lactate decreased, showing that oxidative metabolism increased. Thus, diltiazem increases oxidative metabolism and at the same time relieves angina.

Nakamura et al. presented clinical evidence on the effects of the calcium antagonist diltiazem in decreasing epicardial ST segment elevation in dogs with coronary occlusion and the development of late ectopic beats, as well as in increasing myocardial blood flow in some chronic ischemic dog preparations. These studies focused on the general anti-ischemic effect of calcium-antagonist agents.

But the action of antianginal and anti-ischemic agents is dependent on their total metabolic environment and, in particular, on the *potassium ion concentration*. In his oral presentation, *Henry*[1] made a critical contribution toward clarifying the mechanism of antianginal agents by classifying them as follows: The first group depends on the prevailing concentration of potassium; the second group of calcium-antagonist agents is not potassium dependent. The first group includes nitrates, hydralazine, theophylline, adenosine, and many other compounds.

Abiko et al. took the question of the metabolic classifications even further. They found that nitroglycerin had different metabolic effects from all the other agents. Apparently, in their anesthetized, open chest preparation, nitroglycerin had direct metabolic effects on the heart and did not act through a peripheral mechanism.

W. Schaper made very important points in relation to the *size of the ischemic zone and the ultimate infarct*. He found that, by various modulations, the oxygen uptake and, hence, the size of the ischemic zone is altered; then development of the whole process is delayed so that the collateral flow can come in to provide a permanent beneficial effect. Thus the collateral flow, the size of the ischemic zone, and the oxygen uptake are all critical, as is the extravascular reserve. Furthermore, he described two important new modifications in the method of assessment of infarct size and of therapeutic intervention. First, the infarcted area (detected histochemically after 90 min of coronary artery occlusion followed by 90 min of reperfusion) is compared with the area of the perfusion bed (i.e., the maximal possible expected infarct size if there is no collateral flow). Thus each infarct size as found is expressed as a percentage of the maximum possible expected infarct size. Second, he suggests that a control ligation–reperfusion experiment could be followed by an intervention ligation–reperfusion experiment. These improvements in methodology will undoubtedly lead to a considerable advance in our knowledge of the effects of anti-infarct agents.

Imai et al. pointed out (as supported by J. Schaper et al.) that it seems an oversimplification to suppose that the total ATP level could govern reversibility or irreversibility. They further stated that there are other metabolic factors, including creatine phosphate, that determine whether there is or is not reversibility in their isolated guinea pig heart model.

The contribution that *Neely* would have made almost certainly would have included the necessity for the careful localization of metabolic parameters in compartments and the necessity for trying to match our overall tissue measurements with changes in the compartment in which that metabolite is active.

Opie and Lubbe put forward reasons for linking a cellular accumulation of cyclic adenosine monophosphate (AMP) to the development of arrhythmias

---

[1] Henry presented a paper on the classification of calcium-antagonist agents at the symposium. This differs from the chapter by Henry and Clark included in this volume ("Protection of Ischemic Myocardium by Treatment with Nifedipine").

in ischemia, but it must be recalled that cyclic AMP will probably turn out to be only one of a long chain of events involved in adrenergic effects.

Gudbjarnason and Hallgrimsson proposed that one could alter membrane properties by altering the composition of membrane phospholipids. Though still a speculation, they suggested that perhaps those membrane phospholipids could regulate the sodium and calcium channels. Diet, epinephrine, stress, and related factors could alter the membrane lipids and thus, in turn, alter electrical properties. These proposals certainly give us a challenging concept to think about.

With respect to the application of these basic studies to patients with ischemic heart disease, *Bleifeld et al.* showed how to overcome the very major difficulties of assessing the effects of intervention on *infarct size* and on the severity of ischemic damage in patients. Not only are such measurements tricky and time consuming, but they also require persistence and great care in the collecting and interpreting of data. The studies of Bleifeld et al. also showed that, in patients with severe coronary artery disease, the effects of nitrates were chiefly peripheral.

What about the *direction for future work?* In addition to the specific studies suggested in the discussions above, future work, in general, should take the following into account: To obtain a better understanding of the effects of antianginal drugs requires (a) a very careful examination of the effects of the drug on the myocardial cells and its subcellular components; (b) the use of sophisticated *in vivo* models to study effects on extracardiac sites; and (c) an analysis of direct drug effects on the metabolism of the arterial smooth muscle cell.

REFERENCES

1. Bing, R. J. (1965): Cardiac metabolism. *Physiol. Rev.,* 45:171–213.
2. Bricknell, O. L., and Opie, L. H. (1978): Effects of substrates on tissue metabolic changes in the isolated rat heart during underperfusion and on release of lactate dehydrogenase and arrhythmias during reperfusion. *Circ. Res.,* 43:102–115.
3. Chance, B. (1976): As cited in: Opie, L. H. (1976): Discussion of effects of regional ischemia on metabolism of glucose and fatty acids. *Circ. Res. (Suppl. I),* 38:I-52–I-74.
4. Feldman, R. L., Nichols, W. W., Pepine, C. J., and Conti, C. R. (1978): Hemodynamic significance of the length of a coronary arterial narrowing: *Am. J. Cardiol.,* 41:865–871.
5. Gevers, W. (1977): Generation of protons by metabolic processes in heart cells. *J. Mol. Cell. Cardiol.,* 9:867–874.
6. Hearse, D. J., Opie, L. H., Katzeff, I. E., Lubbe, W. F., van der Werff, T. J., Peisach, M., and Boulle, G. (1977): Characterization of the "border zone" in acute regional ischemia in the dog. *Am. J. Cardiol.,* 40:716–726.
7. Jackson, G., Atkinson, L., and Oram, S. (1977): Improvement of myocardial metabolism in coronary arterial disease by beta-blockade. *Br. Heart J.,* 39:829–833.
8. Jennings, R. B., Hawkins, H. K., Lowe, J. E., Hill, M. L., Klotman, S., and Reimer, K. A. (1978): Relation between high energy phosphate and lethal injury in myocardial ischemia in the dog. *Am. J. Pathol.,* 92:187–207.
9. Kübler, W., and Spieckermann, P. G. (1970): Regulation of glycolysis in the ischemic and anoxic myocardium. *J. Mol. Cell. Cardiol.,* 1:351–357 (1970).
10. Nachlas, M. M., and Shnitka, T. K. (1963): Macroscopic identification of early myocardial infarcts by alteration in dehydrogenase activity. *Am. J. Pathol.,* 42:379–405.

11. Opie, L. H. (1976): Effects of regional ischemia on metabolism of glucose and fatty acids. Relative rates of aerobic and anaerobic energy production during myocardial infarction and comparison with effects of anoxia. *Circ. Res. (Suppl. I)*, 38:I-52–I-74.

12. Opie, L. H., and Thomas, M. (1976): Propranolol and experimental myocardial infarction: Substrate effects. *Postgrad. Med. J. (Suppl. 4)*, 52:124–132.

13. Simonsen, S., and Kjekshus, J. K. (1978): The effect of free fatty acids on myocardial oxygen consumption during atrial pacing and catecholamine infusion in man. *Circulation*, 58:484–490.

14. Steenbergen, C., DeLeeuw, G., Barlow, C., Chance, B., and Williamson, J. R. (1977): Heterogeneity of the hypoxic state in perfused rat heart. *Circ. Res.*, 41:606–615.

15. Whalen, D. A., Jr., Hamilton, D. G., Ganote, C. E., and Jennings, R. B. (1974): Effect of a transient period of ischemia on myocardial cells. I. Effects on cell volume regulation. *Am. J. Pathol.*, 74:381–398.

16. Winbury, M. M., Howe, B. B., and Weiss, H. R. (1971): Effect of nitroglycerin and dipyridamole on epicardial and endocardial oxygen tension—Further evidence for redistribution of myocardial blood flow. *J. Pharmacol. Exp. Ther.*, 176:184–199.

Subject Index